new vital oils

'Liz has always been committed not only to a natural approach to cosmetics but to the importance of beauty from the inside out. *New Vital Oils* is likely to become the definitive guide to which oils we need for our diet and for our skin – and why.'

Kathy Phillips, Associate Editor (Health and Beauty), Vogue

'Liz Earle's specialist research is second to none. This book makes fascinating reading and is guaranteed to have you (not to mention the rest of the family) looking and feeling great in no time.'

Eve Cameron, Editor, She Magazine

'Liz's passionate, knowledgeable approach to all aspects of natural beauty is always inspiring.'

Jenni Baden Howard, The Daily Telegraph

new vital oils

the ultimate guide to radiant beauty and health

LIZ EARLE

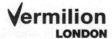
Vermilion
LONDON

For P.J.D
thank you

5 7 9 10 8 6 4

First published in the United Kingdom in 2002
by Vermilion, an imprint of Ebury Press
Random House UK Ltd.
Random House
20 Vauxhall Bridge Road
London SW1V 2SA

Random House Australia (Pty) Limited
20 Alfred Street, Milsons Point, Sydney,
New South Wales 2061, Australia

Random House New Zealand Limited
18 Poland Road, Glenfield,
Auckland 10, New Zealand

Random House (Pty) Limited
Endulini, 5A Jubilee Road, Parktown 2193, South Africa

Random House UK Limited Reg. No. 954009
www.randomhouse.co.uk
Papers used by Vermilion are natural, recyclable products
made from wood grown in sustainable forests.

A CIP catalogue record is available for
this book from the British Library.

ISBN: 0 09 187669 9

Typeset by seagulls
Printed and bound in Great Britain by
Mackays of Chatham plc, Chatham, Kent

contents

acknowledgements

Producing a book is always very much a team effort and I should like to express my most sincere and grateful thanks to all those who have helped to create *New Vital Oils*. I am indebted to the many people who spared their time and generously shared their brain-power on this both complex and fascinating subject. I'm also grateful to the very talented team at Liz Earle Cosmetics and to all those who helped support both my research and me during the lengthy writing process. In purely alphabetical order, special thanks to:

Dr David Atherton, Sue Beechey, Jim Binning, John Black, Kim Buckland, Jacqueline Burns, Joanna Carreras, Jonathan Daniells, Patrick Drummond, Bruce Duckworth, Dr Udo Erasmus, Dr Frances Fewell, Juan Vincente Gomez Moya, Ray Gransby, Madeleine Hewitt, Valerie Holmes, Professor Jonathan Hadgraft, Patrick Holden, Geraldine Howard, Jan Kusmerick, Dr Peter Lapinskas, Dr Roger Leysen, Miren Lopategui, Anna Macleod, Professor Colin Ratledge, Dr Ray Rice, Dr Alexandra Richardson, Craig Sams, Stephen Simmonds, Sarah Stacey, Michael Skipwith, Dr Martin Watt and Rob Williams.

about the author

Liz Earle is known first and foremost for her passion for promoting natural beauty, health and wellbeing. A television broadcaster and best-selling author of many books specialising in beauty and health issues, she is also the creator of the popular Naturally Active Skincare botanical beauty range.

Keen to encourage the dialogue between conventional and complementary medicine, Liz co-founded the UK Guild of Health Writers in 1996 and was the Guild's first Vice-Chairman. She was a co-founder of the Food Labelling Agenda (FLAG), which campaigned at government level for clear, comprehensive and meaningful food labelling. She is also an active member of the Soil Association and an advocator of organic farming and animal welfare. Over the years, Liz has established links with many botanical, dermatological and nutritional research projects, at institutions that include Great Ormond Street Hospital for Sick Children, St Mary's hospital, Portsmouth, The Royal Botanical Gardens at Kew and Greenwich University. She is a Patron of the National Eczema Society.

More information and regular botanical research updates can be found at www.lizearle.com

introduction

When *Vital Oils* was first published in 1991 it helped to break new ground on the importance of oils and fats in our diet. At that time, 'low-fat, no-fat' was the cry and many of us cut out all oils and fats from our daily foods, often with disastrous consequences. (Depression, heart disease and chronically dry, scaly skin are just some of the many unwelcome side-effects of a fat-free regime.) As we now know, not all fats are bad and some are absolutely *vital* for our beauty and health. In fact, after many years of extensive research, I am convinced that *vital oils* in the diet are the very key to our inner vitality and outer radiance.

Today, much more is known about the importance of a group of substances called essential fatty acids (which I shall refer to as EFAs throughout this book) and the many different kinds of oils and oil supplements now widely available. For example, when I first began my research and writing in the 1980s, evening primrose oil was a rare and precious substance. Today, it is one of the world's most popular beauty and health supplements for women, with countless documented clinical trials to support its help for dermatological and hormonal problems. Similarly, although cod liver oil was popular, no one yet knew of the enormous number of benefits that the special fats in this and other fish oils can bring.

Investigations into EFAs are one of the fastest growing and most exciting areas of nutritional research today. Many university and hospital departments run clinical trials covering an astonishingly wide range of ailments and diseases. Some of the most exciting work

1

centres on a special group of EFAs that have been proven to help with depression (perhaps even post-natal depression) and Attention Deficit Hyperactivity Disorder (ADHD) in children and teenagers (see p.33). More effective – and certainly cheaper – than prescription drugs, with the added benefit of no side-effects, they are literally life-changing.

Perhaps the only problem with including these *vital oils* in our diet is the confusing array of supplements and overwhelming amount of information available. Deciding how much, of which oils, to add is a daunting task. Walk into any health shop and aisles crammed with bottles of oils and jars of capsules, each one promising the elixir of life, instantly surround you. Did you know, for example, that evening primrose oil can help hormonal hot flushes, borage oil may help infantile dermatitis, fish oil can help with hyperactivity and conjugated linoleic acid may even speed weight-loss? Information abounds – but the facts are sometimes confusing! The aim of this completely new and comprehensively updated edition of the original *Vital Oils* book is to demystify the different sorts of oils and their uses; and to debunk the more outlandish and unsubstantiated claims, while still singing the praises of some of the finest supplements we have for overall wellbeing.

I hope you will find this book both an interesting read and a useful reference source for the future. Plant and fish oils offer so very many beauty and health benefits that it would be a shame to miss out on what they have to offer. Technical talk about EFAs can, however, be complicated (and boring), so I have tried to remove both the confusion and the jargon – while still leaving in enough to satisfy the sceptics. For this reason most of the technical data has been put at the back of the book, to study, skim or skip as you choose. I have deliberately avoided listing the endless scientific and clinical references, as they would take up a further volume of print. However, they are freely available on many websites and details of how to access them can also be found at the back of the book. In the Useful Resources section (p.201) you will also find many further reference points for more technical detail than this book allows.

Why vital oils?

Natural oils have been described as the 'life force' of a plant and many are famed for their healing properties. Oils from plants, nuts and seeds have played an important part in many ancient cultures, both as powerful medicines and effective beauty treatments. They are also an amazingly concentrated source of vital nutrients that include vitamins, minerals and – most important of all – a group of substances called essential fatty acids (EFAs), required by every living cell in the body to function properly. A lack of these EFAs can lead to many of the ailments associated with modern life, such as stress, heart disease and even cancer, while low levels can lead to many beauty problems, including a dry, flaky complexion, weak nails and dull, brittle hair. Our eating habits have changed dramatically over the years and many of us, without a doubt, now risk a deficiency of these vital oils. In addition, modern food processing has stripped many of these oils of their naturally healthy assets, robbing us of the important nutrients that ensure good looks as well as health.

This book is about replacing this loss of nutrients – and achieving long-lasting health using natural oils. And by health, I mean not just a lack of disease, but a positive feeling of wellbeing – a renewed vitality and zest for life. By taking just a few drops of these golden liquid healers you can not only minimise the risk of many serious diseases and degenerative disorders, but also improve your mood, balance emotions and reduce your risk of depression – and all with no side-effects.

Just like the original version, this book asks you to increase the amount of oils in your diet by a small amount, but (much more importantly) it also emphasises the great care needed when choosing oils. Because it is the *type* of oil that is so vitally important. Oils provide energy and nutrients such as vitamins and EFAs, but not all oils and fats are created equal. Some, such as the saturated fats from animal sources, are unhealthy and should be kept to a minimum. By reducing these, and increasing the amount of plant and fish oils – the *vital oils* – in your diet instead, you can expect to notice a vast difference in the way you look and feel. Here are just some of the many significant health benefits *vital oils* can bring:

○ Increased energy levels, performance and stamina
○ Greater resistance to heart disease
○ Improvement in inflammatory disorders such as arthritis
○ Improved mental agility and protection against depression
○ A stronger immune system
○ Healthier infant and child development
○ Improved vision, wound recovery and healing
○ Clearer skin, shiny hair and strong nails
○ Fewer PMS and menopausal symptoms
○ Better digestion and elimination
○ Reduced allergy symptoms

Many years of research and experience have led me to the conclusion that all these benefits are easily achievable by using the *vital oils* mentioned in this book. Whatever your age, sex or medical history, by including just a few drops of these potent healers in your life every day, you can expect to feel fitter, be less stressed and begin to enjoy a complexion that positively glows with good health and radiance.

1

vital oils:
an overview

In recent years, no single area of our diet has changed more radically than the type of fats and oils we consume. In an attempt to combat heart disease, lose weight and become generally fitter we have moved away from high-fat foods, increased our intake of low-fat products and in some cases, cut out fat altogether. The next time you are in the supermarket, cast your eyes over the huge array of low-cholesterol and fat-free products and you will soon realise the amazing culinary revolution that has taken place on the shelves. The terminology is bewildering, too, with words like 'polyunsaturated' and 'hydrogenated' littering the labels. The wording 'high in polyunsaturates' leads us to believe that a product will somehow be good for us, but is this really true? How many of us truly understand the terminology and its implications for our health? I will admit to being still slightly baffled by the bewildering array of biochemical labelling. That's why I'd like to use this section of the book to explain (and in some cases explode) some of the myths perpetrated by the food industry – most notably, the notion that fat-free diets are healthy – and to explain why certain kinds of oils have so many fantastic benefits for our wellbeing.

Face the fats

In an ideal world we would get all our vitamins, minerals and essential fats from a perfectly balanced diet – i.e. one containing the correct amount of nutrients needed by the body to function effectively. These include fats, proteins, carbohydrates, vitamins and minerals, which should, as far as possible, come from unprocessed, natural foods. By cutting down on certain fats, such as those in some vegetable oils, we run the risk of being deficient in vital substances such as EFAs, which can lead to significant health problems. Essential fatty acids are, as their name implies, *essential* for good health. When first discovered, EFAs were incorrectly called vitamin F because it was thought that they were vitamins. We now know that they are important substances in their own right, although this collective name is still occasionally misused. EFAs are important for keeping the body tissues in good condition and are vital components of the membranes that surround every living cell. The body can't make its own supplies of EFAs so we need to get them from food. This does not, however, mean investing in a deep-fat fryer or welcoming back the daily fried breakfast. It is the *type* of fat in the diet (rather than the quantity) that is fundamental to maintaining a high level of health and glowing good looks.

The structure of fats is a complex biochemical issue. Those who are interested in the science should skip this section and read Fats and oils: the inside story, p.191. For the simpler explanation, see below.

Fats and oils: good and bad

Although all fats and oils look the same, they can vary chemically in ways that can profoundly affect our health. Depending on the number of hydrogen atoms they contain (see p.192), fats can be saturated or unsaturated.

Saturated fats are mostly of animal origin, as in red meat and dairy produce, and are the easiest to identify as they tend to be solid at room temperature (for example, lard, butter and cheese). The excep-

tions to this rule are coconut and palm oils, both from the plant kingdom and both also high in saturates. These two are termed oils, since
in the countries where they are produced the climate is warm, so they
are liquid. In our cooler northern climates they are normally solid fats.
The reason we are advised to avoid this type of fat is because a diet
high in saturates will increase the 'bad' form of cholesterol, the so-
called low-density lipoprotein (LDL), which encourages deposits in
the arteries and raises the risk of heart attacks and thrombosis.
Saturated fats are also bad news because they block the health-
enhancing properties of other, more beneficial types of fats.

Unsaturated fats are considered to be the most beneficial to
health. Depending, again, on their structure (see p.192) they can be
either monounsaturated or polyunsaturated. Monounsaturated fats
are found in plant oils such as olive, rapeseed and avocado. Many
nutritionists consider them to be neutral, which means that, while
not clogging up the arteries as saturated fats do, they do not provide
many extra benefits to health.

The healthiest fats of all are the polyunsaturates, which fall into
two main types, or families: omega-3 and omega-6. (You may also
see these written on supplement packs as ω-3 and ω-6) These two
families differ from each other in only tiny ways (the position in the
chain of the special 'double' bonds) yet the difference is quite criti-
cal to our bodies. The families are totally separate from each other
and cannot be converted from one to another. Both are indispensa-
ble to our health and since we cannot make them for ourselves, they
must be supplied in small amounts in the food we eat. That's why
they are called *essential fatty acids*, or EFAs.

The omega-3 and omega-6 families are found in oily fish and
vegetable oils. Oily fish contain the most significant levels of omega-
3 polyunsaturates, although some forms of omega-3 do come from
vegetable sources, such as flax. The omega-6 polyunsaturates are
found primarily in vegetable oils such as sunflower seed, sesame and
safflower seed oil. We will examine each group and their many
health benefits in more detail later.

Perhaps the greatest good news about polyunsaturated fats is the protection that they can give us against the Western world's biggest killer – heart disease. Omega-6 polyunsaturates, such as sunflower or safflower oil, are believed to do this by reducing the levels of 'bad' cholesterol, or low-density lipoprotein (LDL), in the bloodstream and are often promoted in low-fat diets. However, there is some evidence to suggest that these omega-6 fats may also have the unwanted side-effect of reducing levels of the 'good' type of cholesterol called high-density lipoprotein (HDL), whose function is to prevent choles-terol deposits from settling in our arteries. It's all a question of balance. The normal ratio of HDL to LDL is thought to be 1:5 (one part of HDL to five of LDL), which means that the HDL has to work hard to carry the cholesterol away from the cells and back to the liver, where it is converted into bile acid prior to excretion. An excess of omega-6 polyunsaturates may disrupt the delicate balance between the lipoproteins, tipping it in favour of the less desirable LDLs. This casts a shadow over the health-giving claims made by the makers of polyunsaturated spreads and cooking oils and has led to heated debates between the food industry and some medics. Perhaps more importantly, though, many polyunsaturated products are highly processed by the time they reach our shopping trolley and this refining destroys many of their benefits. The omega-3 polyun-saturates, provided in fish oils, are a far better option as they can give us so many important health benefits, without any of the risks, and we shall look at these in greater detail later, in Chapter 2. For a list of cooking oils divided according to types of fat see p.59.

The cholesterol connection

Polyunsaturated oils are a relatively new discovery, yet in the last 50 years our consumption of them has increased three-fold. As you will see, while this is good news for the makers of highly refined margarine and cooking oils, it is less encouraging for our health.

So how did the polyunsaturates become so popular? The story for their success relates largely to cholesterol, the waxy substance that has been closely linked with heart disease. Cholesterol is used in the body as a component of the membranes surrounding every living cell. Its function is to ensure that the fats we need to transport can be moved around in the largely water-based fluids such as blood and lymph. Cholesterol also helps keep our nerve fibres in good condition and is needed for the manufacture of hormones. Because cholesterol is important to us biologically, the body is capable of making its own supplies, which it does in the liver, and the less cholesterol we eat, the harder our liver works to replace it. So no matter what we spread on our bread, it is impossible to cut cholesterol out of our lives altogether. Not only is it impossible to cut out cholesterol, but it would be highly unwise to do so, as cholesterol is an essential biochemical that the body cannot do without. However, the food industry has latched on to the idea that it is the main culprit when it comes to heart disease. This is simply not true. More accurately, it is the oils and fats that have been damaged by food processing that may be causing us the greatest harm.

Damaged fats

Food processing, such as over-refining and hydrogenation (in which healthy vegetable oils are 'hardened'), converts healthy unsaturated oils to unhealthy saturated fats. These damaged fats are known as 'trans fats' and are found in many commercially prepared foods such as processed meals, 'fast foods', cakes, biscuits and artificial butter spreads. Many studies have linked our consumption of trans fats to a much greater risk of developing heart disease and certain kinds of cancer as well as many other degenerative diseases.

While cholesterol can cause similar problems to trans fats and clog up our arteries – like limescale furring up pipework – the problem cholesterol causes is not entirely due to the substance itself. An unwanted build-up of cholesterol is simply a symptom of the body not being able to process its blood fats correctly, and this again comes down to the type of oils in the diet. The only way to ensure you have a healthy balance of blood fats that encourages the formation of high-density lipoproteins (HDL) or 'good' cholesterol, is to cut down on saturated fats and to limit the use of highly refined fats (such as processed foods and some low-fat spreads). Watch out for any ingredients termed 'hydrogenated', 'hardened' or 'trans fats' on the label. These overprocessed products are damaging to health. Unfortunately, food-labelling law does not currently require the declaration of trans fat contents. However, in practice, manufacturers of products with low levels usually say so on the label, so if the trans fat level is not stated on the label, you can assume that it's significant (i.e. higher than 1–2 per cent).

Fortunately there are many readily available healthy alternatives to trans fats, including the *vital oils* from the omega-6 and omega-3 fat families. In their raw, natural and unrefined state, plant oils such as sunflower and sesame seed, as well as the fabulous fish oils, are packed with health benefits. These oils are all polyunsaturated and have the ability to regulate the delicate balance of lipoproteins. By using them in cooking, we can prevent an excessive amount of LDL from forming, while maintaining or even increasing levels of the beneficial HDL. In addition, fish oil supplements have also been found to be extremely useful for lowering the overall level of fats in the bloodstream and reducing the risk of death from heart attacks.

So although there are many different kinds of fats, only two groups are *essential*. These are the omega-6 and omega-3 fats. All the other fats are termed by nutritionists non-essential because the body can make them for itself. As for the omega-6 and omega-3 fats, we *must* obtain these from our diet to build better health and well-being.

Getting the balance right

Many things in life are a matter of balance and polyunsaturates are no exception. The ratio between the omega-6 and omega-3 group of fats is very important and should be between about 2:1 to 5:1 (i.e. two to five parts of omega-6 for every one part of omega-3). Unfortunately, scientists are not yet agreed on what the exact proportions should be, but what they do agree on is that the current UK and US ratios of 10:1

and 12:1 respectively are too imbalanced in terms of omega-6 fats. This imbalance has arisen because, since 1900, our consumption of the omega-6 fats has increased about 20-fold due to eating so much refined vegetable oil in processed foods. As this has increased, so, too, our consumption of the omega-3 fish fats has dramatically decreased, to about one-sixth of what we were eating 100 years ago. This means that although we need both omega-6 and omega-3 fats, we are not getting anything like the proper balance. In Australia the ratio can be as high as 25:1, as this nation eats little fish yet consumes high quantities of processed vegetable oils.

Having looked at the overall picture of fats and oils, the rest of this book will aim to help you and your family strike the right balance for maximum health benefits. Remember, by choosing just a few drops of the right *vital oils*, you can enjoy better health, every day.

oils for health

'God in His infinite goodnesse and bounty
hath by the medium of plants, bestowed
almost all food, clothing and medicine upon man.'
Gerade's *Herbal* (1636)

Over the years, the medical profession has become increasingly aware of the benefits of oil supplements and a staggering array of capsules and golden liquids now fills the shelves of chemist and health food shops. But despite the recent focus of attention, taking a daily dose of oil to ward off various ills is nothing new. The Ancient Greeks and Romans used olive oil, for example, to heal scar tissue and sunburn by rubbing it on to the body and scraping it off using a curved wooden blade called *strigil*. (The British Museum has an example of two *strigils* standing in a bronze oil pot, used by Roman athletes after athletic training sessions.) Both Pliny and Hippocrates also prescribed it for all kinds of weird and wonderful ailments, from insomnia to boils.

Cod liver oil is the biggest selling oil supplement today, with over 100 million cod livers processed each year in the UK alone. But other supplements from the sea have also caught the eye of the medical world – namely, the oils extracted from the flesh of fatty fish such as mackerel and herring. These oils contain the fatty acids EPA (eicosapentaenoic acid) and DHA (docosahexaenoic acid) required by the body to make prostaglandins – hormone-like substances which lower the likelihood of heart disease by reducing the risk of blood clots forming in the body. Fish oils are also vitally important for healthy brain cells and can be helpful in cases of hyperactivity and depression, proving once and for all the old wives' tail about fish being good for the brain.

Another supplement to arouse particular medical interest is evening primrose oil, which contains GLA (gamma linolenic acid) and also influences the production of a group of biochemical messengers called eicosanoids that transmit genetic information from DNA to cells in the body. Evening primrose oil is one of the most versatile natural healers ever discovered. There is a wealth of scientific evidence to show that it can improve pre-menstrual syndrome, eczema, breast pain and even hyperactivity in children, all of which will be discussed in greater detail later.

Quackery or cures?

The alternative health care industry has more than its fair share of charlatans and quacks, so how can we be sure which oils really are good for our health? After all, the claims are far-reaching and can sound far-fetched. One way to confirm that a substance has been thoroughly researched is to check its medical pedigree. In the UK there are three categories of legally recognised medicines. The first is known in the trade as a GSL, an abbreviation for the General Sales List given to pharmacists and chemists. GSLs are licensed by the Department of Health for specific ailments; for example, cod liver oil has a product licence for relieving symptoms of arthritis such as joint aches and muscular stiffness. The next step up is the P product – this stands for Pharmacy Only and must be sold by, or in the presence of, a qualified pharmacist. Some fish oil capsules have a Pharmacy Licence and may be dispensed to patients with heart disease to relieve symptoms of hypertriglyceridaema (raised levels of blood fats). The final category is POM, or Prescription-Only Medicines and these are only available on prescription. Certain brands of evening primrose oil may be prescribed for the treatment of atopic eczema and, more recently, for breast pain.

Before a remedy can qualify for any of these categories the Department of Health must first be satisfied that it is likely to work for the patient. This involves a lengthy process of double-blind clinical trials carried out under the strictest medical supervision. Half of those tested are given a placebo or dummy set of capsules (usually filled with liquid paraffin), and no one taking part knows whether they are getting the placebo or the real thing, making the point that some patients will improve no matter what they are given! The doctors involved in double-blind trials are also kept in the dark about which participants receive the placebos. This is especially important in cases where the doctor needs to make an impartial judgement on the patient's progress. Clinical trials may take years to complete and it is only when conclusive results have been achieved that a product can be considered for licensing. The fact that so many oil supplements have passed this rigorous procedure is proof that they really can and do work.

The healing oils

Edible oils are naturally enriched with nutrients that improve the way we look and feel. Some, such as olive oil, can easily be incorporated into our daily diet, while others, such as the fish oils and evening primrose oil, come in capsule or liquid form and can be swallowed as supplements. Many have the power to relieve acute ailments such as heart disease and atopic eczema, but all have the ability to improve energy levels and vitality. Plant oils have been used as natural healers for thousands of years and many can be traced back to the Ancient Greeks and Egyptians. Today, scientists are able to analyse their unique chemical structures and can identify the active ingredients in each oil. And although most plant oils look the same, once inside the body they behave in very different ways.

The following guide details the edible oils most readily available to us and is followed by a useful remedy finder designed to help you with specific disorders.

An A–Z guide of healing oils

ALMOND OIL (*Prunus amygdalus*)

Background: The almond tree is a native of the Middle East and now flourishes in the warm, sunny climates of the Mediterranean and California. It was first brought to Britain by the Romans and can be traced back to Biblical times. The Rod of Aaron mentioned in the Bible is thought to have been a branch from the almond tree and twigs of almond blossom are still carried in some Jewish festivals. There are two varieties of tree, the sweet almond (*dulcis*) and bitter almond (*amara*) and both varieties flower in January with a profusion of frothy white blossom. The almonds form on short branches and are protected by a tough outer husk that resembles a greengage. Because of this fleshy covering, almonds belong to the same fruit family as peaches and apricots, although their pulp is nowhere near as tasty. When the almonds are harvested the outer case splits open to reveal the nut inside. Cold-pressing the kernels yields up to half their weight in oil.

Science: The term almond oil almost invariably refers to the sweet variety as this is the one most widely used. Bitter almond oil is not sold to the public as it contains traces of amygdalin, which can be hydrolised or distilled to produce deadly hydrodyanic acid (cyanide). Sweet almond oil is highly nutritious, being a good source of nutrients such as trace minerals and the essential polyunsaturate linolenic acid. It is also a useful source of linoleic acid. In its raw state immediately after extraction, almond oil is a pale yellow colour. However, it usually undergoes an extensive bleaching and refining process that makes it colourless and also reduces some of its nutritional value.

Benefits and uses: Almond oil is a good source of monounsaturated fatty acids (see p.7) and its most recent role is in the prevention of heart disease. Researchers in the USA have found it to be twice as effective as the better-known olive oil in reducing the build-up of cholesterol. Clinical trials published in the *American Journal of Clinical Nutrition* report that after just four weeks on an almond-based diet, the participants' cholesterol levels dropped by an average of 11 per cent. Other control groups taking part in the study included those on an olive-based diet, whose cholesterol levels dropped by an average of 5 per cent, and those on a saturated fat diet high in butter and cheese, whose cholesterol levels not surprisingly increased. Those on the almond diet ate natural almonds and ground almonds and were only allowed to use almond oil for cooking. As a result of this data, the Almond Board of California has urged Americans to use almonds at every culinary opportunity, from sprinkling ground almonds on to yogurt or waffles for breakfast to extending chicken casseroles with these nutritious nuts. Almond oil could also be used in recipes instead of other monounsaturated oils such as olive oil, but would be more expensive. The pharmaceutical industry is a major buyer of almond oil and it is used as a base for ointments as well as in mild laxatives.

BORAGE OIL (*Borago officinalis*)

Background: The Romans called borage the 'herb of gladness' and used an infusion from its leaves to treat depression. Originally from Aleppo in Syria, borage is now grown all over Europe. It is easily recognisable in the herb bed by its bright blue flowers and rough greyish-green leaves. Although borage is not especially aromatic, it attracts bees to the garden and has the nickname 'beebread'. Its flavour is similar to that of cucumber and it is a traditional addition to cold drinks such as Pimm's in the summer. During the Middle Ages, borage was a popular anti-inflammatory agent and was also used to treat rheumatism and heart disease. The 17th-century English herbalist, Nicholas Culpeper, was ahead of his time when he described borage seeds as being useful for increasing supplies of breast milk, as borage has only recently been identified as some of the richest sources of gamma-linoleic acid (GLA) – the essential fatty acid required by babies and naturally present in mother's milk.

Science: Borage (or starflower) is probably best known as an alternative to evening primrose oil. As a result of the research into the medicinal effects of evening primrose oil and its essential fatty acids, scientists began to search for other natural sources of GLA. Both borage and blackcurrant seed are very rich in this important EFA. In fact, borage seeds contain over twice as much GLA as evening primrose oil. The good news for consumers is that because of this, we may only need half as much of it to achieve the same effect. This means swallowing fewer capsules, which should, in theory, cost less. However, although borage is probably a very useful supplement (especially for the skin) there is considerable debate over whether it is as beneficial as evening primrose oil for other reasons.

Benefits and uses: The main medical benefit of GLA is helping to control the inflammatory response in conditions such as eczema. We'll look at this further on p.46, but basically it's all to do with the regulation of substances called prostaglandins. Although borage oil is high in GLA, it does not appear to have the same action as GLA on the specific prostaglandins that help regulate inflammation. So, although borage oil is a very useful supplement for general skin health and maintenance, it is wiser to choose evening primrose oil when looking to treat specific disorders such as eczema.

COD LIVER OIL

Background: Physicians used cod liver oil to treat rheumatism and gout as long ago as the 18th century, when it was naively thought that the oil benefited the body by lubricating the joints. Dr Samuel Kay carried out some of the first medical experiments involving cod liver oil in 1752 at the Manchester Infirmary. He used it to treat bone disorders and rheumatic pain, and it later became widely used for diseases relating to malnutrition, such as rickets. The medical profession accepted that cod liver oil worked, but no one knew just *how*. Today we know that its health benefits come from the fat-soluble vitamins A and D, together with high levels of polyunsaturated fatty acids (PUFAs).

Cod liver oil does literally come from the liver of cod, most of which are caught in the North Atlantic waters around Iceland and Norway. Deep-sea trawling is a laborious business and involves sinking nets 190 fathoms deep over an area several miles long. The nets are hauled in two to three hours after dropping and the fish swim up to the top of the net where their escape is blocked with a knot. This is called the Cod End – hence the trawlermen's expression, 'It all comes out of a cod end.' The cod has an unusually large liver and it can take just ten livers to produce one gallon of oil. In the old days, the fish was landed and cleaned on the quayside and the livers tossed into large oak barrels, where they were left to rot. After a period of days, or even weeks, the oil would ooze out from the liver cells as they disintegrated – and we can only imagine the stench. As the oil floated up to the top of the barrel, it was skimmed off and strained, ready for bottling.

The oil produced in this way was a dark, evil-smelling brew and sold mainly to the tanning industry for softening leather hides. It was a small, but lucrative, sideline for the trawlermen, who treated the proceeds as pin money. This changed in the mid-1850s when cod liver oil was found to be an effective cure for rickets. This debilitating childhood bone disease causes bowlegs and tragic malformations of the joints and is due to a lack of vitamin D. During the Industrial Revolution it was common amongst the children of the workhouses, who spent much of their undernourished lives working in appalling factory conditions. Charles Dickens powerfully portrayed the plight of these children and there is no doubt that Tiny Tim would have benefited from a daily dose of cod liver oil.

When doctors discovered that cod liver oil could prevent and even cure rickets, the demand soared. It became clear that simply leaving the cod livers in barrels to rot was an inefficient means of production. So the steam extraction process was developed, which involved boiling up the livers in huge vats and siphoning off the oil. These vats were fitted into the cargo holds of the trawlers and to compensate for the extra workload the fishermen were paid liver money. Cod liver oil production became big business – and caused intense competition amongst the fishing fleets. This rivalry finally ended for one group in the 1930s when several fleet owners in Hull got together and decided that their time would be better spent working with, and not against, one another. They formed the British Cod Liver Oil Producers Ltd (later re-named Seven Seas), a co-operative that marketed the oil and passed the proceeds back to the men on the boats.

At about this time vitamin D was identified for the first time and found to be present in cod liver oil, and at last doctors began to understand one of the reasons why the supplement is so valuable. Later, when food rationing was in force during and after the Second World War, the Ministry of Food organised free distribution of cod liver oil to all children under five, and to pregnant and breast-feeding women, to prevent malnutrition. After the war, the Welfare Foods Scheme decided that this should continue as, despite the rigours of rationing, Britain's war babies were the healthiest the nation had ever seen.

Although we think of rickets as a disease from the past, some races in Britain remain at risk even now. These include the large Asian communities who have settled in Glasgow, Birmingham, Manchester and Leeds. In addition to obtaining vitamin D from our diet, we also synthesise it through our skin when it is exposed to sunlight. Although the feeble British sunshine suits the fair-skinned British, darker-skinned races have more difficulty absorbing enough to make vitamin D. This is a particular problem for Asian communities, as they tend to cover themselves up more when outdoors (especially women and girls). The result can be a serious vitamin D deficiency, and this has led to a worrying resurgence of rickets amongst Asian children. The Department of Health has launched a campaign to make the Asian community more aware of the risks to their children and is once again advocating the use of cod liver oil.

Since its discovery, many more health benefits from cod liver oil have been identified, and what was once the trawlerman's sideline now rivals the catch itself in terms of importance.

Science: The main nutrients found in cod liver oil are vitamins A and D. Both are stored in the fat cells of the liver and are said to be fat-soluble. Vitamin D regulates growth and also improves the tensile strength of teeth and bones by controlling calcium absorption. While the body can manufacture some of its own supplies through the skin, this amount can need supplementing. The richest sources of vitamin D are (in order) halibut liver oil, cod liver oil, herring, mackerel, salmon and sardines. Vitamin A is an important nutrient for healthy eyes, skin and hair and for building our resistance to respiratory infections. Because the vitamins in cod liver oil are retained by the body and stored in the liver, it should not be taken in vast quantities, which could be potentially hazardous. This is especially important during pregnancy, when excess vitamin A should be avoided.

Benefits and uses: Cod liver oil is one of only a handful of dietary supplements to be granted a medical licence. In this case it is for relieving the pain caused by aching joints and muscles. But to assume that the oil works by simply lubricating the joints is somewhat of an over-simplification. Cod liver oil contains the omega-3 polyunsaturated essential fatty acid, used by the body for the production of useful substances such as eicosanoids, prostaglandins and leukotrienes. Leukotrienes are similar to prostaglandins in that they control functions such as blood pressure and the digestion, but they also regulate inflammatory disorders. The level of leukotrienes in the body must be carefully balanced, however. Too many leukotrienes can result in their instructing cells to begin harmful disease processes such as blood clots and inflammation. Cod liver oil is able to regulate the leukotrienes, making it a very useful supplement in the battle against inflammatory disorders such as arthritis (see Arthritis, p.37) and inflammatory kidney disease, in which the omega-3 fats have been shown to reduce the need for kidney transplants and minimise the need for dialysis.

One of the best-known cod liver oil enthusiasts of this century was American laboratory technician Dale Alexander, otherwise known as the Cod Father. His passion for this amber nectar stemmed from the fact that it cured his mother's painful arthritis, and *Arthritis and Common Sense* was the first of five books he wrote on the subject. The Cod Father advocated a tablespoonful of cod liver oil a day mixed with milk to disguise what he called its three flavours: 'ucky, yucky and bloody awful'. The first scientific paper published on cod liver oil and arthritis appeared in a 1959 edition of *The Journal of the National Medicine Association*. This described a study where 98 patients were given 20ml (4 teaspoons) of cod liver oil mixed with milk or orange juice taken on an empty stomach. A 92 per cent success rate in relieving pain and swelling was recorded, with many patients also noticing an improvement in the condition of their hair, skin and nail condition. It was also noted at the time that part of the success of the oil might have been due to its being taken on an empty stomach. Subsequent double-blind clinical trials carried out at Albany Medical College in New York during the 1980s also confirmed cod liver oil's effectiveness at relieving morning stiffness and tender joints.

Cod liver oil has also been successfully used to treat many inflammatory skin conditions and researchers are currently exploring other inflammation disorders, including asthma (see Asthma, p.38). A poor supply of omega-3 fats is also thought to be a contributory factor in allergies and this is another area of nutritional medicine with ongoing research.

The recommended daily dose of most cod liver oil supplements is 10ml (2 teaspoons), although some health practitioners suggest increasing this to 20ml (1 tablespoon). One of the best ways to take cod liver oil is to emulsify it by shaking it together with a small amount of milk or fruit juice before drinking. This helps to break down the oil into tiny droplets that enable the digestive system to process it faster. Shaking it with another liquid in this way kick-starts the process that occurs naturally later on in the liver. Another advantage is that it helps to avoid the 'fishy breath' that can occur after swallowing the liquid or capsules, especially if taken on an empty stomach. Emulsified fish oil supplements are also now widely available for this reason. When buying fish oil supplements, choose a reputable supplier such as Seven Seas, which carries out stringent quality control checks for pollutants, or choose supplements that specifically say they are extracted from deep sea fish oils, such as Nutri.

Of course, there is far more to fish than cod liver oil and health benefits can be found in every form of fish – from a sardine sandwich to the latest fish oil supplements. We grow up to believe that fish is good for us, yet few of us know exactly why. Amidst the mass of generally accepted folklore sits the theory that fish feeds the heart and brain, and there is increasing scientific evidence to support this belief. Fish oils thin the blood, so reducing the risk of blood clotting. They have also been linked to increased mental energy and play a vital role in brain development. There is an enormous amount of scientific evidence to support their help for the brain, from treating Attention Deficit Hyperactivity Disorder (ADHD) and dyslexia in children to clinical depression, schizophrenia, autism, Huntingdon's disease and more besides (read more on some of these specific disorders on p.33). Clinical trials to date are promising. One American study with people suffering from severe manic-depression had to be stopped early because the results were so good for those taking fish oils that it would have been unethical to withhold them from the control group! Sophisticated brain imaging, carried out at one of London's leading teaching hospitals in Hammersmith, is also showing unprecedented reversal of brain damage in mental patients taking the supplements. There seems to be little question that these specific *vital oils* can dramatically improve brain function.

Brain food and beyond

Fish oils are rich in the fatty acid DHA – the main polyunsaturate found in the thinking part of the brain. About a quarter of the dry weight of our brain is made up entirely from DHA, making it hugely important for all of us. DHA is also used in quantity to make up the retina of the eyes and to help build healthy nerves. The first studies found that rats raised without DHA in their diet had offspring that were less mentally alert. DHA is vitally important for human intelligence too. We know that there is an enormous surge in DHA levels in the brain of an unborn child during the last three months of pregnancy. Some scientists suggest that babies born prematurely may be at risk of incorrect brain development due to DHA deficiency and baby milk manufacturers have been urged to increase the amounts of DHA in feeds made especially for premature babies. You'll find more about this important area under Pregnancy and Babycare, p.53.

Over the last decade, fish oils have been subjected to close medical scrutiny, since the discovery that they are able to alter the balance of blood fats in the body. This is another important attribute of the polyunsaturated omega-3 essential fatty acid group. The only organisms to manufacture their own plentiful supplies of omega-3 EFAs are the single-cell plankton that live in the depths of the ocean. These marine algae are now being explored as a food supplement and added to foods such as margarine. All fish contain a certain amount of these essential fatty acids simply because plankton is their main source of food and so the omega-3s are stored in their fat tissue. However, oily fish from cold waters such as herring and mackerel are a far better source than white fish such as haddock or plaice. Further up the food chain, seals and whales also have high levels of omega-3s as their diet consists entirely of fish. And the Inuit, who live largely on whale and seal blubber, are one of the few races to have a diet that is naturally enriched with these essential fatty acids. This is believed to be the main reason why they have such a low rate of heart disease and strokes.

Fish oil supplements can go rancid relatively quickly, so don't bulk-buy and always keep them in the fridge. Brands vary, so if you find that one type doesn't suit you, it's worth trying another make before dismissing them all. Cod liver oil is a good source of omega-3 fats but it also contains high levels of vitamin A, making it less suitable for small children and for use during pregnancy. Fish oils generally have few side-effects but they do act as blood-thinning agents, so talk to your doctor before taking them if you are also using blood-thinning medications such as daily aspirin or Warfarin. Because of their ability to thin the blood, fish oils should not be taken for a couple of days before planned surgery and those with diabetes should also discuss this with their doctor as very large doses may raise blood sugar levels. Most fish oil capsules contain around 250mg oil per capsule, but daily dosage is very much a matter of personal choice. Diabetics should not take more than 2000mg a day without first consulting their doctor.

Eat more fish!

You won't need to take fish oil supplements to prevent heart disease if you eat oily fish at least twice a week. Reducing the amount of harmful triglycerides simply means eating more fish oil and this can be done through delicious fishy foods. In the past, fish was plentiful and cheap and was a major part of the average Briton's diet. In the 18th century, masters were actually taken to task for making their apprentices eat salmon every day. But one thing the nation did not suffer from was heart disease. Nowadays, we eat far less fish and the types we do eat, such as cod, haddock and plaice, contain the least amount of oil. When choosing which to eat, opt for for the darker, fleshier varieties such as herring and mackerel as these contain more of the omega-3 fats.

Tragically, although eating more fish is a dietary recommendation for almost every country in the world, global fish stocks are steadily depleting, and fishing communities all over the world are experiencing dramatically reduced catches. This is largely because huge trawlers drag the sea-bed with enormous, tight-weave nets that gather up every living thing, leaving the sea bed like a desert. So many fish are taken that not enough are left to breed. The trawlers leave nothing for the remaining fish or other sea creatures to eat – and kill up to half of what they do catch because many sea creatures and baby fish are not wanted. The rape of the seabeds by trawlers has been likened to the destruction of entire forests; only nobody actually sees it happening. The answer for those who want to eat fish with a clear conscience is to buy from sustainable sources. (See Useful Resources, p.201). Those who simply can't stand the thought of regularly eating oily fish can supplement their diet with fish oils (or flax oil as a vegetarian alternative). Look for the wording 'pure fish oil' on the package as this should mean that the oil has not been overly processed and that the basic structure of the important omega-3s has been preserved.

Since writing the first edition of *Vital Oils* more than a decade ago, it has been interesting to see the UK government recommendations for our weekly intake of fish oil double from 1.5g to 3g per week. This is the equivalent of one to two portions of oil-rich fish per week, depending upon the variety, and will provide us with 2–3g of the long-chain essential fatty acids. These recommended amounts are increased three-fold during pregnancy but avoid large amounts of cod liver oil during pregnancy due to its high levels of vitamin A. Some experts suggest we should all be aiming for 500mg of fish oil per day, as this is the level that has been shown to be effective in increasing protection against heart disease. Anyone suffering from high blood pressure, arthritis or psoriasis may need higher amounts – possibly 2000–3000mg per day. Eating more fish increases total polyunsaturate levels, too, which means that more protective anti-oxidants (particularly from fat-soluble vitamin E) will be required to keep the polyunsaturates stable. So a daily natural-source vitamin E supplement should also be considered. To find out where the best sources of omega-3 fats can be found, see the omega-3 content chart on p.195.

EVENING PRIMROSE OIL (*Oenothera biennis*)

Background: The evening primrose is a tall, spiky but elegant plant that only blooms in the evening, hence its common name. It is not really a primrose at all, but a spindly wild flower more closely related to the garden flower godetia, and also the rosebay willow herb. Its origins can be traced back 70,000 years to its first appearance in Central America and Mexico. Although evening primroses often grow alongside rivers and streams, these vivid yellow flowers can also be found flourishing in the desert. North American Indian medicine men were the first to recognise the healing potential of evening primrose and brewed the seed pods to make an infusion for healing wounds. They also made poultices from the leaves to soothe aches and sprains and used the juice from its roots as a cough mixture. Later adopted by herbalists, its leaves were used to make mild disinfectants, sedative and diuretics. The Romans also respected its powers and early trans-lations from Pliny state, 'it is an herbe good as wine to make the heart merrie. Of such virtue is this herbe that if it be given to drink to the widest beast that is, it will take the same and make it gentle.' In 1650, the English herbalist Nicholas Culpeper also records his use of the evening primrose, saying 'It opens obstructions of the liver and spleen, provokes urine, is good for the dropsy if infused in common drink.' (Dropsy is the old-fashioned word for oedema, or swelling, and is not a disease in itself but a sign of kidney or heart failure.)

Traditionally called the King's Cure-All, over 1000 different types of evening primrose plant have now been identified worldwide. According to geologists, the evening primrose colonised North America at least four times – narrowly escaping extinction during successive ice ages. It was officially bought to Britain by the English naturalist John Tradescant the younger in the late 17th century. He called it the Yellow Herb of Virginia and it was subsequently re-named the Tree Primrose. Later, towards the end of the 18th century, the newly established trade routes between North America and Europe brought many more of the seeds to Britain. These seeds were stowaways aboard the many merchant ships, which were loaded with extra ballast for stability in the form of stones, sand and soil. The soil contained evening primrose seeds, which germinated and colonised the coastline close to where the ballast was eventually discarded. The flowers can still be seen growing here alongside the coastline of Liverpool.

Unusually for a wild plant, the genetics of the evening primrose species have been the subject of scientific study for well over 100 years. Investigations into this fascinating herb began in 1860, when it was discovered that *Oenothera* hybrids do not follow the usual routes of genetic inheritance. These findings put forward a theory of mutation and the origin of a new species. This botanical curiosity was the forerunner of much of the medical research we benefit from today. The genetic science is complicated, but, essentially, as long as the plant genes remain the same, the activity of the plant is preserved. If hybrids are made, this could inactivate some of the delicate mechanisms within the plant. This has serious implications for farmers who grow evening primrose as a seed oil crop and it must be hoped that cross-pollination as a result of genetic modification will not destroy one of our most valuable nutritional medicines.

Science: In addition to its impressive history the evening primrose continues to gather accolades and medical attention now focuses solely on the oil-bearing seeds of this remarkable plant. The seeds themselves were first analysed in 1919 and found to be rich in fatty acids, including one in particular, identified for the first time as gamma linolenic acid (GLA). Its composition was found to be about 90 per cent unsaturated fatty acids of which 9 per cent is GLA. It was at about this time that the concept of EFAs was identified and their importance in our diet recognised. We now know that these nutrients are needed to maintain healthy body tissue and are also important components of the membranes surrounding every living cell.

As the body has difficulty making enough of its own GLA, we need to obtain extra supplies from the foods we eat. Useful sources include vegetables (especially the green, leafy kind), vegetable oils (especially certain seed oils) and pulses. These foods all contain small amounts of linoleic acid that the body can convert into GLA. However, in many people this vital process is blocked by a build-up of saturated fats, trans fats or highly processed cooking oils or margarines. Poor nutrition may also be a factor, as the conversion process also requires the presence of other nutrients such as vitamin B6, zinc and magnesium. Health problems such as diabetes, viral infections and hormone changes including pregnancy and the menopause can also block much of the conversion, and the process can also be hindered by factors such as old age, alcohol and smoking. However, as these EFAs are so vital for good health it is very important that the body either converts sufficient supplies or receives supplements from an enriched source such as evening primrose oil. To emphasise the importance of EFAs, the World Health Organisation (WHO) advises that EFAs should make up at least 3 per cent of our total calorific intake and that this should increase to 5–6 per cent for children and breast-feeding women. In fact, one of the few sources of GLA itself is human breast milk, a substance renowned for its nourishment and ability to protect the immune system.

The gamma linolenic acid found in evening primrose oil is biologically important as it affects much of the enzyme activity in our body. Every process that takes place within us is triggered by the action of various enzymes, including the production of prostaglandins – hormone-like substances which regulate bodily functions including blood pressure, digestion and inflammation. The Swedish scientist U.S. Von Euler discovered them in the 1930s, in the prostate gland, and so named them prostaglandins. Since then, around 40 different prostaglandins have been identified and occur in every cell in the body. Prostaglandins regulate the movement of material between individual cells, control cell-to-cell communication and the transmission of signals between nervecells. Although biochemists have yet to pinpoint exactly how all prostaglandins work at a molecular level, these hormone-like substances seem to exercise control over just about anything and everything in the body. Unlike hormones, though, prostaglandins are not secreted from glands in the body and then transported to where they are needed. Instead, we are able to produce them on the spot in response to a stimulus anywhere in the body. Also unlike hormones, prostaglandins live for only a few seconds before being broken down, which is why we need a steady supply of GLA to ensure our prostaglandin levels remain stable. Their action as regulators and internal messengers means they have a dramatic affect on overall health and each year literally thousands of medical research papers are recorded involving prostaglandin activity.

Benefits and uses: Because of the effect evening primrose oil has in boosting our GLA and thus prostaglandin levels, this natural supplement has been the subject of a record amount of interest around the world. Diabetes is just one disease currently under investigation using evening primrose oil therapy. Diabetics suffer from a blockage in the process that converts linoleic acid into GLA. Exactly why this occurs is not yet clear, but it seems to be linked to an imbalance of metabolic hormones and prostaglandins that regulate the release of insulin. However, initial double-blind clinical trials show that diabetic nerve damage can be repaired with 4000mg of evening primrose oil, taken every day for a six-month period.

Other clinical trials are also currently underway to assess the effect of evening primrose oil on inflammatory disorders, such as osteo- and rheumatoid arthritis and irritable bowel syndrome. Encouraging results of evening primrose oil therapy have also been seen in cases of alcohol-induced liver damage, hyperactivity in children and cystic fibrosis. Evening primrose oil may also have a stimulating effect on converting fat into energy and could be useful in treating obesity and discouraging general weight gain. In addition, impressive results have been reported when it is used for disorders associated with hormonal imbalances – a great number of women suffering from pre-menstrual syndrome (PMS) have found evening primrose oil capsules useful for reducing the symptoms of bloating, water retention, irritability and depression.

Many women already take a daily capsule or two of evening primrose oil to ward off such ailments. However, to help improve many of the more acute conditions described over the following pages, the dose must be increased to 2000mg to 4000mg every day for a minimum of four weeks. The ongoing medical interest in evening primrose oil will no doubt ensure that, whether used as an all-round tonic or a specific treatment for more serious disorders, this humble herb plays an increasingly important role in our health protection and wellbeing.

FLAX (LINSEED) OIL (*Linum usitatissumum*)

Background: Flax (or linseed) oil takes its name from the Latin word meaning 'most useful' and comes from the flax plant. Flax is an annual crop with rich blue flowers and tiny brownish-yellow seeds. There are several different varieties, each with different uses. The long-stemmed variety is grown for its lengthy fibres that are woven into linen, while the short-stemmed varieties tend to concentrate their goodness in the seeds, used for oil extraction. Flax needs a rich, wet soil with plenty of hand labour and is an important crop in Northern Ireland where it is used to make traditional Irish linen. The oil-laden seeds are warm-pressed to extract the oil and several organically grown varieties are available in most health shops.

The use of linseed oil as a healer can be traced back to Hippocrates, who recorded that it was a useful treatment for stomach and skin disorders. More recent advocates of linseed oil include Mahatma Gandhi, who wrote, 'Whenever flax seed becomes a regular food item among the people there will be better health.' Indeed, ancient Indian writing dictates that to reach the highest state of contentment and joy, a *yogi* must have a daily dose of flax oil. Linseed has traditionally been valued by herbalists for its mucilaginous properties, meaning that it contains a slimy material that is not absorbed but passes straight through the body. Linseeds are a very effective and gentle bulking agent and can be used as a laxative when swallowed whole with plenty of water. The mucins and water-binding substances in the linseeds work by increasing the volume of the stool within the bowel. This then presses against the intestinal walls and triggers the action of peristalsis (intestinal movement). In addition, the mucins form a protective and gliding film that covers the sensitive mucous membranes. This can help heal any intestinal wall irritation and can be very helpful in cases of constipation or irritable bowel syndrome.

Crushed linseeds are also used by herbalists in poultices as they have the ability to draw out excess fluid from body tissues. Linseed poultices are sometimes used in this way to treat the swollen fetlocks of racehorses and even help heal human athletic injuries. Some aromatherapists also use linseed poultices in conjunction with massage to help temporarily tighten slack skin tissues and combat cellulite. Today, the overwhelming use for flax or linseed oil is as an additive for paint manufacturers and it is also sold as conditioning oil for cricket bats. However, following the discovery of its essential fatty acid content, linseed oil is making a timely nutritional come-back.

Science: Of all the seeds used for oil extraction, linseeds give up their oil with the least struggle and the oil accounts for over half their weight. Although a relative newcomer on the health food market, linseed oil (or flax as it is more commonly referred to for food use) contains mainly omega-3 and some omega-6 fatty acids. The oil is a particularly rich source of the omega-3 alpha linolenic acid which can, to some extent, be converted by the body into EPA and DHA –

the long-chain omega-3 polyunsaturates found in fish oils. Linseed oil has therefore been recommended as a useful alternative for vegetarians who prefer not to take fish oils. However, research has shown that this conversion process in the body may be limited. For this reason it is important not to overlook the extraordinary value of the omega-3 fish oils. In addition to its high levels of essential fatty acids, flax oil also contains the antioxidants beta-carotene and vitamin E.

Benefits and uses: According to the oils-for-health specialist Dr Udo Erasmus, flax oil provides the best therapeutic source of omega-3 fats because it contains the largest amount of alpha-linolenic acid. He points out that this EFA helps disperse deposits of saturated fats, such as cholesterol, which like to make our blood platelets sticky. A unique factor is that flax oil is thought to contain a substance similar to prostaglandins that help regulate hormone activity within the body, which may in turn help to improve our immune system. Unrefined flax oil also contains lecithin and other phospholipids that help emulsify other fats and oils within the body, so easing digestion.

Flax oil has been used therapeutically by many complementary practitioners for several decades. Some of the most extraordinary reports come Dr Johanna Budwig, a West German biochemist and nutritionist, who claims to have successfully treated many cancer patients with flax oil. Budwig has long believed in the use of unrefined oils to promote good health and help heal serious diseases. Her unusual dietary regime involves taking 120ml (8 tablespoonfuls) of flax oil in 100g (4oz) of cottage cheese every day. Dr Budwig's theory is that the sulphur-rich proteins in the cottage cheese help ensure that the EFAs in the oil are utilised properly in the body. She says: 'It is obvious that if we feed the body the highly unsaturated essential fatty acids it requires, along with the high quality protein which makes the fat easily soluble, and if we also stay away from chemical preservatives, then many, many people will become healthy very fast. I have proved this premise many times.' Dr Budwig claims to have over 1000 documented cases of successful cancer treatment using flax oil and her controversial work has been repeatedly nominated for the

Nobel Prize in medicine. However, with such a difficult and emotive disease as cancer, it is clear that more research needs to be carried out to assess the true value of this kind of nutritional therapy. For further in-depth information, read *Fats that Heal, Fats that Kill* by Dr Udo Erasmus (see Further Reading, p.212).

One of the drawbacks to flax oil is that it needs to be used fresh as it spoils much faster than other oils. Even when kept cool and slightly sealed, it loses many of its nutrients after just four months – light, air and high temperatures destroy its omega-3 alpha linolenic acid very rapidly. Flax oil should therefore be kept in the fridge and used within six weeks of opening. However, the oil is also available in capsule form, which protects the oil longer from spoilage. When buying the liquid oil, choose one that has been packed in a light-proof container, such as a black plastic bottle or tin. Because of its short shelf life, the best varieties carry both the date the oil was extracted *and* a best-before date. It must be said that flax oil has a peculiar 'organic' taste and is best used in blended salad dressings or added to flavoured milkshakes. It can also be combined with other oils such as olive and sunflower oil to boost their nutritional value.

the healing oils
remedy finder

While increasing the amount of *vital oils* in your general diet will improve overall health and vitality, many health problems will need specific treatment with oil supplements. Below is an alphabetical resource of ailments and conditions that can be treated with *vital oils*. For more information on each problem and relevant support groups see Useful Resources, p.201.

Attention-deficit/hyperactivity disorder (ADHD)

Attention-deficit/hyperactivity disorder is now one of the most common childhood diseases. Together with dyslexia (specific reading difficulties), dyspraxia (developmental co-ordination disorder) and the entire autistic spectrum, it represents one of the main challenges to juvenile mental health. All relatively common (and on the increase), these conditions have a high degree of overlap and have significant implications not only for the children and families affected, but also for our whole future society. It is estimated that up to 20 per cent of the British population may be affected to at least some degree by one or more of them. Pharmaceutical drugs are often the first lines of treatment, but they are expensive, often ineffective and can leave lasting side-effects. Taking food supplements of EFAs may well be helpful and is certainly a safer choice than some drug-based therapies as there are no adverse side-effects.

Ritalin is an amphetamine drug taken by millions of children worldwide to treat ADHD. In recent years it has become one of the most commonly prescribed medications for young children living in the Western world. However, many have voiced their concerns and fears over its rising use. While the drug certainly calms and subdues affected children, it can also cause sleep problems, stunted growth and a depressed appetite. American researchers have shown that Ritalin has a similar effect on the brain to cocaine. Brain scans of 11 healthy men who took a child's dose of Ritalin showed that the drug blocked 70 per cent of the dopamine transporters that remove excess dopamine from the system (cocaine typically blocks about 50 per cent). Dopamine is the chemical messenger that sends 'pleasure' messages to the brain that an experience is worth repeating. If little dopamine is able to reach the brain, this may be the reason why typically fun activities don't give ADHD children much pleasure. It may also explain why some drugged-up children become almost robotically placid. Studies in the respected *Journal of Neuroscience* have also shown that children with ADHD who take Ritalin may be more prone to drug addiction in later life.

In the search for safer medication for young children, many researchers are turning their attention to nutritional therapies and several specific *vital oils* are showing great promise. Dr Alexandra Richardson, Senior Research Fellow in Neuroscience at the Imperial College School of Medicine at Hammersmith Hospital, London, is certain that the increasing amount of 'junk' food is a contributory factor in many children's mental health problems. She believes that taking the drug Ritalin should be a last resort rather than a first line of treatment and that nutritional supplements will help some children with ADHD, dyslexia and dyspraxia. In her studies of groups of children with these three conditions, Dr Richardson charted the progress of those given omega-3 and omega-6 supplements and those given a placebo (a dummy supplement). The EFA supplement contained three important fats: EPA, DHA (from fish oils) and GLA (from evening primrose oil). In every instance the placebo group showed no improvement while the others performed better in speech and movement, co-ordination, vision and writing, levels of aggression and impulsive behaviour. When the placebo group was given the EFA supplements, it too made sudden and similar progress, a crossover that convinces Dr Richardson her findings are accurate. Interestingly, other symptoms were relieved by the EFA supplements, too, including excessive thirst, frequent urination, dry and rough skin (especially around the tops of arms and thighs), brittle or soft nails, dry hair, dandruff and a wide range of inflammatory conditions.

I know from first-hand experience just how helpful some of the *vital oils* can be for distracted children. My own young son is class-ically dyslexic, with poor short-term memory and low concentration. I have found significant improvement in both his behaviour and abil-ity to concentrate when he takes his daily spoonfuls of fish oil and evening primrose oil. I have recommended this *vital oil* therapy to several friends with 'disruptive' children, each time with great success. One mother of a four-year-old notoriously 'wild' child reported a very significant improvement in his behaviour after giving him a simple daily fish oil supplement. Another friend with a teenage son called to say that both she and her son's teachers had seen a dramatic change for the better in his behaviour within four days of taking fish oil! She has seen not only improvements personality-wise within the family at home, but also a marked improvement in his schoolwork and class reports. I know yet another man who grew up with dyslexia, becoming clumsy, uncoordinated with poor concentration and short-term memory. The experts were gloomy, he was listed for a special needs school and his mother was warned to expect a difficult, disruptive teenager. Fortunately, she had heard of other mothers in the USA giving their dyslexic children large quant-ities of fish oils and it seemed to work for her son. So great was his improvement she now wryly reports that his doctors say he must have been misdiagnosed … So instead of reaching for the Ritalin, my overwhelming advice is to try this simple, inexpensive and often highly effective nutritional therapy first.

Vital oils are not just for young children. They have also been linked to helping aggressive behaviour in adolescents. Japanese research with young adults who have high levels of fish oil in their daily diet has found that when stress levels are raised (for example during college exams), their likelihood of aggressive behaviour is reduced. It seems that the EPA and DHA in fish oils may act as a regulator of mood and emotion when we are stressed. A low level of DHA in the brain may explain why some of us are more prone to random acts of aggression, such as road rage. Further nutritional studies amongst prisoners have found that the most violent offenders tend to have the lowest levels of EPA and DHA within their brains.

As yet, scientists have not been able to pinpoint precisely how much, and of which, EFAs are helping to improve proper brain functioning in children and young adults. There seem to be no universal answers and our own unique constitution, metabolism, dietary needs and habits make it difficult to create one rule for all.

For proper brain function, the omega-3 fats seem to be more important than the omega-6 family, with probably equal emphasis being placed on EPA and DHA (although expert opinions differ). However, the GLA from evening primrose (and possibly borage and blackcurrant seeds) is also likely to be of some benefit. The current wisdom is to consider supplementing mainly with fish oils but that many people may also benefit from adding in a dose of evening primrose oil. It is a case of trying various combinations and seeing what works for you and your family. Any combination of these *vital oils* is likely to bring very real improvements to other aspects of health and wellbeing too, so there is little to lose and a lot to gain.

It is important to remember that although improvements can be seen in some children in just a few days, it can take up to three months for the maximum benefits to be fully realised. This can be due to the slow turnover of the fatty acids within the brain. Unlike prescription drugs, they do not work by rapidly changing mental functioning and changes may be frustratingly slow and gradual. In terms of dosage, again there are no hard and fast rules. The acknowledged expert on this subject, Dr Alexandra Richardson, suggests a higher dose for the initial three-month 'trial' period. An initial dosage of fish oil supplying around 500mg daily of EPA (considered to be the most important fatty acid in this particular case) is probably the best for dyslexia and related conditions, with 50mg per day of GLA from evening primrose oil. After three months is up, you could try reducing this dose to one-half or one-third of these levels. However, Dr Richardson advises that dosages are often determined from personal experience and careful monitoring and that some may need high levels on a long-term basis to prevent symptoms from reappearing. If no improvements are noticed within three months, then it is unlikely that a fatty acid deficiency is a factor in the condition.

Arthritis

There are so many health benefits associated with EFAs – especially the omega-3 oils – that they have been linked to just about every serious chronic ailment. Patients with rheumatoid arthritis (and, according to the latest research, also possibly osteo-arthritis) as well as other conditions resulting in sore and inflamed joints have been found to benefit especially from high doses of fish oils. While these can't re-build degenerated cartilage, bone or synovial membranes they can be highly effective at reducing pain and inflammation. Many studies published in specialist arthritis and rheumatology medical publications have shown that both omega-3 and (to a lesser extent) omega-6 oils can be helpful, especially when substantial doses are taken daily.

Many conditions involve the body's process of inflammation and rheumatoid arthritis is probably one of the commonest. Rheumatoid arthritis is a condition of long-term, chronic inflammation and is an auto-immune disease, which means it is triggered by the body's own immune system. The body's immune system starts to attack itself, leading to damage and inflammation to the tissues of the joints, making them swollen and extremely painful. Finding a substance that will reduce the rate of inflammation is one of the best ways to solve the problem of this inflammatory disorder.

Fish oils (and, to a lesser extent, the same omega-3 fats found in flax, walnut and rapeseed oils) can help, as they are naturally rich in eicosanoids – substances which can help to reduce inflammation and pain, swelling and tissue damage within the body. Studies of rheumatoid arthritis show that supplements of omega-3 fats, such as fish oils, can reduce pain and the morning joint stiffness associated with the disease. This is why cod liver oil has a medicinal product licence and is able to make claims relating to help for arthritis on its packaging. In addition to providing practical help, some studies show that taking regular fish oil supplements also reduces the need for anti-inflammatory drugs. Nutritionists tend to suggest quite a high daily intake of about 6000mg a day when treating rheumatoid arthritis. In this case, you may find the fish oil supplements easier to take if you divide them into separate doses, for example, 2000mg taken three times a day with meals. Initial trials in rheumatoid arthritis have indicated that evening primrose oil may also help bring relief from symptoms, allowing patients to reduce the dosage of conventional medication (and their associated risk of side-effects), so a daily dose of this *vital oil* might also be a sensible addition. Alternatively, a study from the University of Massachusetts Medical Center has shown that very high doses of the essential fatty acid GLA, this time from borage oil, reduced damage to joint tissue in those with rheumatoid arthritis. Taking 240mg of GLA a day resulted in less joint pain and subsequent swelling.

Asthma

Just like arthritis (see above), asthma is an inflammatory condition, except that in this case it's the delicate linings of the lung that become inflamed, affecting breathing. Again, as in arthritis, it is the reduction by the eicosanoids of the inflammatory processes within the body that may be helpful. Early studies indicate that daily omega-3 supplements may have a role to play in helping to reduce this type of inflammation and could, in theory, be of benefit. Some asthmatics report an improvement in their symptoms after taking a daily dose of cod liver oil for some weeks. However, for some unknown reason, fish oil supplements have not been helpful for asthmatics who are also sensitive to aspirin. More research is needed – and indeed is slowly starting to happen. If this condition affects you or your family, it is worth keeping an eye on the medical papers relating to EFA and nutritional therapies published on various specialist websites. More details can be found under the Useful Resources section on p.201.

Breast pain

Pre-menstrual breast tenderness is another complaint that can respond well to *vital oils*, this time by treatment with evening primrose oil. Women with mastalgia (severe breast pain) can now obtain a standardised form of GLA, extracted from evening primrose oil, on prescription from their doctor. Many breast conditions are governed by the action of hormones and breast growth is stimulated during the teenage years by hormonal activity. By their early twenties, most women have reached their final bust size, although almost all will notice slight changes in breast shape and texture during their monthly cycle. It is quite common for breasts to enlarge in the two weeks before a period, and to return to normal after the period begins. A much more visible change takes place during pregnancy when hormones can double breast size and increase blood flow by 180 per cent. While these hormonal fluctuations are perfectly normal, some trigger other breast problems.

The most common breast disorder is pre-menstrual mastaglia, which affects some 5 million women in Britain between the ages of 20 and 50. Other benign (non-cancerous) breast problems include nodularity or lumpiness of the breast just before a period, and fibroaidenomas – smooth movable lumps most often seen in young women. But breast pain is the commonest complaint and can affect either part or the entire breast and even extend to the upper arms.

Women with breast pain are unusually sensitive to hormonal actions. This increased sensitivity is linked to the pattern of EFAs in the bloodstream and these women often have low levels of GLA. They may also have high levels of saturated fats that increase the effects of hormones on breast tissues and trigger pain. The first experience of mastalgia can cause the terrible fear of breast cancer. Fortunately, breast pain is rarely a symptom of cancer and is also far easier to treat. However, conventional medications are far from ideal. Painkillers and diuretics are frequently ineffective and hormone-related drugs carry their own side-effects. In an attempt to find a more acceptable, natural cure for breast pain, double-blind clinical trials involving evening primrose oil were carried out at the Breast Clinic of the University of Wales in Cardiff. Here, pharmaceutical quality evening primrose oil was compared to the most commonly prescribed drugs for this condition, Bromocriptine and Danazol. All three medications were similarly effective, but their levels of side-effects differed enormously. Only 2 per cent of women given the evening primrose oil experienced any side-effects at all, compared to 23 and 25 per cent per cent for Bromocriptine and Danazol respectively. Also, the side-effects for those taking the evening primrose oil formulation were much less acute, the most common being a mild stomach upset. The medical team from the Cardiff clinic reported in the *Lancet* that, after reassurance about cancer, evening primrose oil treatment should be the first line of medication for breast pain. Their studies found that 45 per cent of women suffering from persistent, severe breast pain benefited from the 300mg dose of evening primrose oil. However, as the oil works by changing the EFA composition of cell membranes, it is inevitably a slow cure and the dose must be taken every day for three to six months.

A word about breast cancer: While evening primrose oil can be effective at treating breast pain, it should not be seen as a panacea for all breast problems. The good news is that preliminary studies suggest that the omega-3 fats found principally in fish oils may help to protect against breast cancer. Researchers at the University of California are looking at using omega-3 fats to help maintain healthy breast tissues and believe there is a possible protective effect against breast cancer. In addition, animal studies have found that fewer breast tumours develop when fish oils are included as part of the everyday diet.

Depression and mental health problems

It is a sad fact that one quarter of the British population (some 15 million people) will, at some time, be diagnosed with some sort of mental health problem. The World Health Organisation (WHO) has predicted that, by the year 2020, depression will be the world's second biggest killer after heart disease. Depression doesn't only kill through suicide, but also leads to an early death in other ways. According to Professor Jeffrey Gray of the Institute of Psychiatry in London, 'Depression changes the structure of the brain and there is evidence linking it to cancer, infectious diseases, premature ageing and dementia.' How appropriate, then, that the two most enormous health problems of heart disease and depression may be helped to a great degree by fish oils.

Danish researchers undertook some of the first research into the link between *vital oils* and depression in the early 1980s. They compared international dietary habits to discover why it was that those in developing countries tended to have less severe cases of depression and schizophrenia, despite poorer medical care. It soon became clear that the higher the intake of omega-3 and omega-6 oils, the more patients improved, whereas the higher the intake of saturated fat, the worse they were.

An annual meeting of psychiatrists in Edinburgh in 2000 highlighted special nutritional needs for schizophrenia, especially with regard to fish oils and antioxidant vitamins. This is because the inflammatory response within the brain of patients may be connected to an imbalance of essential fats. Giving daily supplements of 10g of concentrated fish oil (in this case a medicinal product called MaxEPA) led to a significant improvement in schizophrenic symptoms. Interestingly, two additional studies have shown that babies destined to become schizophrenic are significantly less likely to have been breast-fed during infancy. And in later life, there is evidence that the amount of certain polyunsaturates in the diet can influence schizophrenic symptoms. Similar findings have been presented for depression, indicating a clear link between EFAs, brain development and mental health. Further studies in Australia have linked the steep national decline in the popularity of eating fish with a sharp rise in the cases of depression.

Human brains need the right 'engine oil' to function properly and, in this case, that 'oil' contains the long chain polyunsaturated fatty acids EPA and DHA. Phenomenally, it seems that we can change the way our brains behave simply by shifting the balance of *vital oils* within the body. Preliminary studies suggest that the omega-3 fats (notably EPA and DHA) may reduce the severity of schizophrenia by about 25 per cent. Subsequent research carried out at London's leading Hammersmith Hospital has shown that it is possible to dramatically improve the brain scan results of schizophrenics following fish oil therapy. Using the most sophisticated brain imaging technology, Professors Graeme Bydder and Joseph Hajnal found that it was possible to reverse the typical shrinking pattern of a schizophrenic patient's brain and actually encourage re-growth. A large-scale study on manic depression started in 1999 at The McLean Hospital in Belmont, Massachusetts, led by Dr Andrew Stoll, was stopped early because the benefit of the fish oil treatment were so marked that it was considered unethical not to give it to all the patients involved! Manic depression or severe bi-polar depression, as it's medically known, affects around one in 100 of us and has increased 100-fold over the last century, except in countries such as Japan, Korea, Malaysia and Taiwan where it remains rare. These are all countries where almost everyone eats a large amount of fish, especially raw fish in the form of *sushi* – raw fish delicacies bursting with beneficial fish oils.

Some of the best news for this nutritional therapy is that it is both safe and free from side-effects. Unlike prescription drugs, which invariably suppress symptoms at a price, essential fatty acid supplements at the very least can do no harm, whereas common conventional medication, such as Prozac, may cause suicidal or homicidal thoughts in some patients as well as depressing libido – one of the very symptoms of depression that it's meant to cure. Nutritional therapy using the essential fatty acids EPA and DHA is gaining ground, with many conventional medics now starting to recognise and acknowledge its benefits. As more articles and studies appear in the major psychiatric journals it is one of the most exciting and significant areas of medical research.

Dry skin

Although not a serious skin disorder, dry, irritated skin is a problem for many that can be easily solved by adding *vital oils* into the diet. In fact, the nutritional significance of EFAs such as GLA was initially highlighted in trials involving animals who were deprived of these oils and fed on a totally fat-free diet. The creatures quickly developed skin disorders, most noticeably very dry, scaling patches of skin. We, too, would see similar skin disorders if we cut out oils from our diet completely, which is one reason why very low-fat and fat-free diets can be so damaging. One of the many functions of the EFAs in our diet is to maintain the water barrier that exists beneath the *Stratum corneum*, or uppermost layer of skin cells. A dry, devitalised complexion is not caused by a lack of oil in the skin, but, rather, to the evaporation of water through this barrier. Therefore any holes or weakened areas in it will allow more moisture to escape and lead to excessively dry skin. GLA is an important constituent of the cellular membranes that makes up this barrier, so we need to receive regular supplies to ensure that it remains stable and strong. Taking a daily supplement of 3000mg evening primrose oil, 1000mg borage oil or 1500mg blackcurrant seed oil will supply around 240mg of GLA and help to protect the skin from dryness and signs of premature ageing.

Eczema

Excessively dry, itchy skin is often the first sign of the more serious skin condition, eczema. The word eczema comes from a Greek verb meaning 'to boil' – a good description of the often inflamed and intensely itchy skin of this distressing disorder. The commonest form of eczema is atopic eczema. It is thought to be triggered by allergies, and commonest in families where there is a history of asthma and hay fever. Atopic eczema is due to a faulty immune system which leads to the body being unable to distinguish invading bacteria and viruses from harmless environmental substances such as pollen, house dust and mite droppings.

Many sufferers are driven to distraction by the overwhelming urge to scratch, which inevitably leads to severe scaling, bleeding and weeping of blisters under the skin. Not only is eczema unsightly, it is also extremely uncomfortable and frustratingly difficult to cure. Although eczema is so common – atopic eczema is now the most common childhood disorder in the Western world – conventional medicine has yet to find a drug that effectively treats the condition without damaging side-effects. Drugs from the doctor's surgery include steroids and antihistamines, which can work for some but they do have side-effects and are often disappointingly ineffective. Atopic eczema is commonest amongst young children and Dr David Atherton, paediatric dermatologist at the Hospital For Sick Children, Great Ormond Street, is in no doubt of the mental as well as phys-ical scars it leaves on the victim. He says 'in some respects it is easier and less distressing to care for a child with leukaemia than a child suffering from atopic eczema. The disease causes unbearable phys-ical distress for which there is often little relief.'

Children who develop atopic eczema do so between the ages of three and six months, at the time when most are weaned. One clue that the gamma linolenic acid (GLA) in evening primrose oil could be a factor in curing eczema was found when breast-fed babies who switched to solids developed the disease. Human breast milk is a rich source of GLA and breast-fed babies receive the same amount of GLA found in two to three capsules of evening primrose oil every day. Although the makers of formula feeds claim their products are as close in composition as possible to human milk, it is surprising that they rarely contain any GLA at all. According to one manufacturer, adding GLA is 'unnecessary and impractical' and would reduce shelf life. However, the Japanese manage to add GLA to their formula milks by a process of micro-encapsulation. British formula milks contain linolenic acid, which should be converted by the body into GLA. However, studies show that some babies do not carry out this conversion process properly. Even purely breast-fed babies may not receive enough GLA to protect them from eczema if their mother's blood has low levels of this important fatty acid. This suggests that it might be sensible for women who are breast-feeding to supplement their diet with evening primrose oil.

Studies show that children already suffering from atopic eczema have unusually low levels of unsaturated fatty acids in their bloodstream. Having established the link between GLA in evening primrose oil and eczema, literally hundreds of trials involving children with eczema have taken place. The department of dermatology at Bristol's Royal Infirmary carried out one of the most widely publicised trials. Results published in the *Lancet* medical journal reported a significant improvement in patients with atopic eczema who took GLA. These improvements were recorded after just three weeks of taking 4000mg of evening primrose oil a day (2000mg a day for children). The evening primrose oil was shown to improve itching by 36 per cent, scaling by 33 per cent and redness by 29 per cent. Similar trials at the dermatology clinic at the University of Bologna in Italy reported 'substantial improvements' in the clinical symptoms of atopic eczema after just four weeks of evening primrose oil therapy.

My own eczema developed when I was a toddler and remained very much with me until my early twenties, when I first discovered the benefits of *vital oils*. There are few conditions more demoralising than serious skin disorders that won't respond to treatment and I didn't hold out much hope as I swallowed my first doses of evening primrose oil. However, the effect was remarkable. Within a few days the itching stopped and my skin started to heal. The roughened, scaly patches that covered my arms began to fade, until after just one month they had disappeared altogether. I have taken evening primrose oil (along with other essential fatty acids) on a regular basis ever since and my eczema rarely returns.

The two main ways in which evening primrose oil can help improve dry skin and eczema is by preventing water loss from skin cells and regulating the inflammatory processes that lead to skin scaling and itching. The key 'ingredient' in the recipe for eczema is prostaglandin E1, a substance that has a number of important actions within the body. Prostaglandin E1 can dilate blood vessels, lower blood pressure, regulate the immune system in response to allergens and have an anti-inflammatory action. Anyone looking to improve the condition of atopic eczema should therefore look closely at ways to improve their levels of prostaglandin E1. Evening primrose oil is an obvious choice as it is a rich source of GLA, which leads to the production of prostaglandin E1. But what about the other sources of GLA, such as borage (starflower) and blackcurrant seed oils? Although these are both good sources of GLA and have useful benefits for the skin, they do not appear to be as good at stimulating the production of this prostaglandin. The reason why is unclear, but it is thought that other fatty acids present in both borage and blackcurrant seed oils may have a negative effect. So, although both borage and blackcurrant seed oils are useful supplements for general skin health and our overall wellbeing, they are probably not the best option for specifically treating atopic eczema.

Evening primrose oil is the only oil to have been granted a medical licence to help treat eczema. It is available on prescription for the relief of atopic eczema in a standardised form called Epogam. As small children find it hard to swallow large capsules, Epogam also comes in capsules with a twist-off neck so the oil is easily squeezed onto food. Bottles of liquid evening primrose oil are also available from health food shops. According to Senior Research Fellow in Neuroscience Dr Alexandra Richardson, tendencies towards certain allergic (or 'atopic') conditions such as eczema, asthma, hay fever and so on seem to be more common in people with dyslexia, ADHD or their related conditions. Low levels of EFAs in the diet can play a role in these allergic conditions and supplementation with fish oils as well as the evening primrose oil can often help to relieve some of the symptoms. The most frequently recommended therapeutic dose for evening primrose oil is 1000mg three times daily. This supplies 240mg of GLA a day. To get the same amount of GLA from other sources you would need to take 1000mg of borage oil or 1500mg of blackcurrant seed oil each day. However, these alternative sources may not be as beneficial for those with certain inflammatory conditions such as atopic eczema.

Eye conditions

Fish oils have a reputation for protecting the eyes as well as the brain. Studies published in the *Archives of Ophthalmology* found that people with macular degeneration (the commonest form of vision deterioration) ate more saturated and processed fats, including margarine, and also smoked more. By contrast, the risk of eye disease was lower for those who ate more omega-3 oils found in fish and some vegetable oils, such as walnut, rapeseed and flax. It has long been shown that these EFAs are important to maintain the health of certain vascular tissues, including those that lead to the retina from the brain. Now it seems that omega-3 oils are important to maintain healthy vision, provided they are not eaten with an excess of omega-6 oils. Again, it is the balance between these vital oils that could be so useful when seeking to improve eyesight and help protect overall ocular health The recommended dosage for the problem is 3000mg a day of fish oils.

Heart disease

It was the Inuit in Greenland who inspired the notion of using fish to treat heart disease, when researchers noticed that the Inuit population rarely suffered heart disease or strokes and had no incidence of diabetes. This finding was unexpected, as seal and whale blubber – both integral parts of their diet – are high in cholesterol, which has been largely linked to heart disease. Genetics were ruled out when it was discovered that when the Inuit moved to Canada and adopted a Western diet, their incidence of heart disease went up to match that of the Canadians. Clearly, something in their Arctic homeland was influencing their health.

Attention focused more closely on their diet, which, despite its high cholesterol content, was also found to be very rich in omega-3s. The omega-3 polyunsaturates were found to have the extraordinary ability of reducing a group of blood fats called triglycerides. While the Inuit were found to have similar cholesterol levels to Westerners, their triglyceride levels were only about a quarter as high. Triglycerides are fat molecules consisting of three fatty acids (hence the name *tri*-glyceride). A high blood triglyceride level has been a known risk factor for heart disease since 1953 when nutritional studies began. Since then, evidence has accumulated to show that high triglyceride levels lead to a higher risk of heart disease.

Cardiovascular disease – by far the leading cause of death in the Western world – covers a number of conditions, including coronary heart disease (CHD), acute myocardial infarction (heart attack) and atherosclerosis (hardening of the arteries caused by fatty deposits constricting blood flow) and stroke. Large amounts of triglycerides in the bloodstream can block the body's natural ability to break down blood clots. This can lead to thrombosis, caused when a clot forms within a blood vessel and blocks the blood supply to important areas of the body such as the heart or brain. Thrombosis can rapidly result in a heart attack or stroke and is the principal cause of death for people in the UK over the age of 45. Fortunately, the omega-3 fats can help reduce the risk of death from cardiovascular disease in two ways: firstly, by reducing the levels of triglycerides in the blood and secondly, by stabilising the fatty deposits in the arteries so they are less likely to rupture. This is a very important point, as the omega-3 fats also increase the elasticity of red blood cells and these cells need to be especially pliable in order to flow freely down the finest capillaries in the body, which are often less than 1mm thick. Red blood cells can be as much as three times the diameter of these tiny blood vessels, but are still able to squeeze through. If the red blood cells lose their elasticity they are unable to reach the surface of the skin, the brain or the heart, and blood supplies to these vital organs dwindle. This can result in life-threatening problems such as heart attacks.

Another way omega-3 fats reduce the risk of heart attack is by improving the blood-clotting mechanism. Blood clots form when components of the blood called platelets stick together and it is the eicosanoids in omega-3 fats that make this less likely to happen. By contrast, the EFAs from omega-6 fats, such as arachidonic acid, make this more likely to occur. The final way in which the omega-3 fats are believed to work is by regulating an abnormal heart beat (arrhythmia). According to Professor Mark Vilquist, Head of Medicine at Monash University, Australia, and Chairman of the Australian Nutrition Foundation, 'People who have fish once a week, let alone probably up to three times a week, are much less likely to die suddenly from abnormal heart rhythms.' Interestingly, in this case it is once again the *balance* between the omega-3 and omega-6 fats within the heart muscle that can affect the risk of sudden cardiac death – and it is the omega-3 fish oils that are helpful in controlling arrhythmias. So important was the overall life-saving discovery of the fundamental link between the omega-3s and heart disease that, in 1982, the eminent British doctor and scientific researcer Professor J.R. Vane was awarded the Nobel Prize for medicine for his work on the subject.

The evidence on help for heart disease is one of the best examples of how the omega-3 group of EFAs can significantly improve our health. Many studies since the 1980s have linked low levels of omega-3 oils with heart attacks and the implication is that eating more fish oils really can help save lives. One more recent 1990s study reported in the *European Journal of Clinical Nutrition* examined the fat tissue stores of 100 people aged 45–75 years who had experienced a first heart attack. All these people were found to have lower levels of omega-3 long-chain fats (p.191) than the control group – and higher levels of trans fats, as well as slightly higher levels of omega-6 and short-chain omega-3 oils. As trans fats are found in dairy foods and many artificially hardened (hydrogenated) vegetable fats such as margarine, processed cakes, biscuits and other long shelf-life foods, while the long-chain omega-3 oils are found principally in oily fish, the dietary message is clear. A further study of 11,000 Italian heart attack survivors found that, after four years, the group who had taken fish oil supplements had 20 per cent fewer deaths, despite the fact that all participants had a healthy Mediterranean diet rich in other *vital oils*, such as olive oil. It seems that these powerful omega-3 fats found principally in oily fish really can and do save lives.

Heart disease is the UK's biggest killer of both men and women – almost one in three of us will die from the disease. However, this appallingly high figure can easily be reduced and there is no reason why any of us should become just another statistic. Checking your level of blood fats is one simple way of detecting if you are at risk. More than half the population of the USA have their blood fats analysed at some time by a simple blood test, yet in the UK the figure is much lower. Pin-prick blood tests are available at many health shops and chemists, or your GP will be able to arrange one for you. A simple way of assessing cholesterol levels is to gaze into your eyes. A raised cholesterol level often shows up as a milky white ring surrounding the iris or coloured portion of the eye. Common amongst the elderly, this early-warning cholesterol ring can show up in those as young as 25 and is a surprisingly accurate form of diagnosis. The recommended dosage for preventing or improving heart disease, or for reducing high blood pressure is 2000–3000mg of fish oils per day.

Multiple sclerosis

Multiple sclerosis affects one in every 1000 people in Britain and most of its sufferers are young adult women. Although the exact cause is not yet known, it is believed to be an auto-immune disorder, triggered when the body's own immune system starts attacking itself.

What sets off this extreme reaction isn't known. Some researchers believe that it may be caused by a virus (possibly even a common one such as measles or Herpes simplex) that has possibly lain dormant for several years. The disease affects the nervous system and begins with the destruction of the protective sheath called myelin that surrounds nerve fibres in the brain and spinal cord. The symptoms of MS include blurred vision and a tingling or numbness in the body, which can sometimes lead to paralysis in later life. These symptoms vary in severity and may come and go from one week to the next, so a patient who is severely disabled one week may seem quite normal the next. While we don't know what prompts MS to strike, we do know that people with MS lack certain essential fatty acids, especially linoleic acid. This deficiency is thought to be an important factor in the degenerative nature of the disease. Studies using evening primrose oil have found its high levels of GLA useful in preventing the immune system's white blood cells from attacking the myelin sheath and destroying the vulnerable nerve cells underneath. Some medics suggest that evening primrose oil may be more active in children suffering from MS and that it may help if given as a protective measure to children in MS families.

Nutritional therapy is often helpful for those with MS, with high doses of antioxidant vitamins as well as the herbal remedy ginkgo biloba to help improve blood circulation. Several EFAs are also recommended, including 10ml (2 teaspoons) of fish oil a day to supply 2g of omega-3 fats. It is suggested that this is combined with 1000mg of evening primrose oil taken three times daily.

A CASE HISTORY

Sue was 29 when multiple sclerosis struck. A previously healthy, energetic and athletic person, her first symptoms were blurred vision and dizziness. She tells the story of what happened.

> I woke up one morning and realised that my eyes wouldn't
> focus properly. When I stood up I felt very dizzy and unsteady,
> and I couldn't control my eyes. My neurologist recommended

taking evening primrose oil from the beginning. My doctor, who luckily for me, is one of the more enlightened medics, also recommended it. I was diagnosed in May 1988, and have been taking six essential fatty acid capsules a day (each containing 430mg of evening primrose oil and 107mg of fish oil) ever since. I have to touch wood before I say that my symptoms have never returned and I can honestly say that I have never felt healthier. I have totally reassessed my diet and don't ever eat any saturated fat. All my oil requirements come from the capsules. I just think that you've got to start thinking about making the cellular insulation material myelin. Taking these *vital oils* provides the essential fatty acids for the body in the form of GLA, which is like giving fat in a pre-digested form. I'm sure that if I stopped taking it my cells would be less protected and I won't take that risk. I feel much better now altogether – even my cellulite has vanished and my skin has a much smoother, more youthful texture. I put it down to my revised diet and would advise any sufferer to seek advice from an informed doctor or qualified nutritionist.

Pre-menstrual syndrome (PMS)

It is thought that about 40 per cent of women worldwide suffer from some form of pre-menstrual syndrome. Many sufferers first experience the symptoms of irritability and depression during their teens, while others escape until their early thirties. It affects all races and levels of society and some of the more famous sufferers include Queen Victoria, Maria Callas, Marilyn Monroe and Judy Garland. One of the main causes of pre-menstrual syndrome is the imbalance between the hormones oestrogen, progesterone and prolactin just before menstruation. An excess of prolactin in particular is linked to high stress levels and has a direct effect on breast pain, causing tenderness and swelling. These three hormones are governed by a group of prostaglandins called PGE1, PGE2 and PGF2, which can cause the uterine contractions that lead to stomach cramps and water retention.

Evening primrose oil is known to affect and regulate the action of prostaglandins and has undergone extensive trials to pinpoint its action in relieving PMS. One such experiment, detailed in the *Pharmaceutical Journal*, took place at St Thomas's Hospital in London. Sixty-eight women took part, all of whom were classed as having severe PMS symptoms that failed to respond to conventional medication. The participants were given 2000mg of evening primrose oil a day (4 x 500mg capsules) and at the end of the trial 61 per cent said they had total relief from PMS, while 23 per cent reported partial relief.

It is believed that PMS sufferers have low prostaglandin levels caused by poor absorption of linoleic acid or an inability to convert it into GLA. By regulating the action of PGE1, PGE2 and PGF2 the oil can then correct the imbalances that can lead to the condition. Early research indicates that evening primrose oil may also be beneficial to women with endometriosis and could even play a role in reversing infertility. Some studies also show that the omega-3 fats found principally in fish oils may be helpful in easing menstrual cramps.

Supplementing your diet with 3000mg a day each of fish oils and evening primrose oil may be a useful form of nutritional therapy.

Pregnancy and babycare

Pregnancy is a time when a mother-to-be invariably pays more attention to her diet and the foods she is eating. This is also a time of life when the omega-3 essential fats are perhaps at their most important. As the developing baby grows, so it draws from its mother a full range of vital vitamins, minerals and essential fatty acids. The omega-3 fats (and DHA, in particular) are especially significant during this time, as they are needed to create body and nerve cells, notably for the eyes and brain. Evidence is increasing all the time to suggest that a rich supply of omega-3s in the mother's diet can help to ensure proper brain and vision function in the child.

Omega-3 intake is especially important during the third trimester, or final three months, of pregnancy as this is when the developing baby needs the additional supplies of DHA most. Later, once the baby is born, he or she still has a high need for both omega-3 and omega-6 essential fats from breast milk. Studies have shown that breast-fed children perform better in cognitive tests than those fed formula milk. There is a vast difference between breast milk and artificial formula milk. Almost all formula feeds are made from cow's milk (with soya or goat's milk alternatives for babies who have problems digesting dairy foods) which is designed to fatten up cows, not humans. Breast milk is especially important during the first few weeks of a baby's life as it contains a special fluid called colostrum, rich in antibodies to build the baby's immune system. Breast milk also contains hormones and human growth factors that simply cannot be recreated in the laboratory. In addition, breast milk is a richer supply of the important essential fatty acids required for all aspects of a new baby's development – especially if the mother supplements her diet with omega-3 and omega-6 fats.

PREMATURE BABIES

For babies who are born prematurely, the issue of how many essential fatty acids they receive becomes even more crucial. These pre-term babies have not yet received the full share of maternal DHA that they were due and there is evidence to suggest that what little they have is not enough to develop their nerve and brain development properly. Tests show that premature babies fed on breast milk (naturally rich in DHA) for at least four weeks have a significantly higher IQ at the age of seven years than a comparable group fed only formula feeds.

POST-NATAL HEALTH

Not only is it important for a mother-to-be to maintain high levels of the omega-3 fats in her diet, but these should be maintained post-delivery too. This is partly so that her breast milk remains a rich nutritional supply for her baby, but also to replenish her own supplies, which will have been given to the developing baby during pregnancy. This is especially important for mothers who have had more than one baby in quick succession, as their stores of omega-3 fats may be replaced too slowly or incompletely for their overall health. A need for the omega-3 group of essential fatty acids doesn't disappear once a baby has been weaned on to solid food either. Interesting studies have found that babies who are the tragic victims of cot death, or Sudden Infant Death syndrome, have had low levels of these polyunsaturates within the brain. It may be that these *vital oils* play an important protective role in infant health too.

As babies develop, so their need for EFAs continues, especially with regard to intelligence and brain development. Researchers at Dundee University have found that babies given a simple task took less time to complete it if they had been fed with fish oils. Dr Peter Willatts, who carried out the research, explains:

> Two groups of babies were asked to complete a series of tasks involving a succession of picture matching. The group given the [fish oil] LCP (long chain polyunsaturate) supplement from birth were measurably faster in finding the correct images. Other intelligence tests showed them to be more efficient in understanding and solving problems.

It has also been found that the eyesight of very young babies who had received these EFAs developed more quickly and comprehensively, possibly leading to better vision, and that enriched infant milk might also be associated with lower blood pressure in later life. In view of so much supporting evidence, the decision to formula-feed is not one to be taken lightly. Breast-feeding is not only safer, more convenient and protects your baby from infection; it also provides the right amount of nutrients at a time when they are needed for vital development. But if you can't (or decide not to) breast-feed, it's especially important to read the label on the formula tin and make sure that the formula is enriched with a good source of the long chain polyunsaturated (omega-3) fats. Whether for mother-to-be or her baby, there is possibly no other time of life when these *vital oils* become quite so vital.

POST-NATAL DEPRESSION

As we have already discovered, some *vital oils*, notably the omega-3 fish oils, can be very helpful in helping to prevent and improve cases of depression. Many studies have shown fish oils to be beneficial, especially when it comes to help for post-natal depression. International studies show that new mothers are 50 times less likely to suffer post-natal depression if they eat plenty of fish. Results published in 1999 by the US National Institute of Health linked data from 17,000 people in 24 countries around the world, in which researchers studied links between the rates of fish consumption and post-natal depression in new mothers. For example, in Japan only 3 per cent of new mums suffer depression and they eat an average of 67kg of fish a year. By contrast, a staggering 20 per cent of all Australian women get the baby blues – and they eat a meagre 19kg of fish on average a year. Cultural factors such as extended families helping out with child-rearing can play a part, but Professor Mark Vilquist, chairman of the Australian Nutrition Foundation believes the link with fish oils to be an important one. He says, 'The levels of omega-3 fish oils is a predictor of mood, so the case for enriching the central nervous system with these fatty acids, and it having a favourable effect on mood, is growing. There is increasing evidence that fish consumption – which only needs to be quite modest in the main – can improve mood.'

Psoriasis

Psoriasis – an often distressing skin condition in which the skin cells renew too quickly, leading to scaliness and flaking – is mainly treated with creams and lotions designed to help slow down the rate of skin cell formation. But as many sufferers will tell you, these are not always effective. Psoriasis, too, has been linked to problems with the metabolism of EFAs. A study of 80 patients who were given omega-3 fish oil supplements showed significantly reduced lesions within four to six weeks. Itching was the first symptom to decrease, followed by scaling, then redness. Essential fatty acids may also help when applied directly to the skin and some natural treatment creams contain specialised EFAs and other helpful oils. One called PS-98 Dermanova contains omega-3 fish oils, neem seed oil (see p.103) and cactus extracts. These ingredients may also be helpful for those with eczema and stockist details are listed at the back of the book in Useful Resources.

In addition to dietary supplements, it is important for psoriasis patients to avoid all damaged, trans fats and to focus on a 'clean food' diet. It may also be helpful to cut back on the saturated fats found in red meats, dairy foods (especially cheese) and eggs, as well as refined sugars and wheat gluten. Some practitioners also suggest milk thistle and artichoke extracts to help improve liver function. Sufferers from psoriasis also seem to benefit from taking evening primrose oil and clinical trials have reported moderate improvements in 60 per cent of patients given 2000mg supplements over an eight-week period. The dosage for omega-3 supplements recommended for treating psoriasis is around 3000mg of fish oils a day.

4

oils for food

'Out of the ground made the Lord God to grow every tree that is pleasant to the sight, and good for food'
Genesis 9:1

All the vitamins, minerals and essential fats we need to eat can be naturally found in the foods that grow on our planet. Nothing needs to be artificially created. Some of the most important foods we have come from plant oils, which appear in our daily diet in many varied forms. You may think that your oil consumption is confined to the frying pan or to salad dressing, but in reality, oil it is far more prevalent in the form of fats. These can account for 40 per cent of our average daily food intake, or more. This is because they appear in almost *all* processed and convenience foods, from the obvious chips and crisps to the hidden fats in meat pies, sausages, hamburgers, cakes, biscuits, ready-meals, pastries, sweets, chocolate, ice-cream, puddings and much, much more. Understanding the way these fats and oils are produced and treated – and knowing how to choose your cooking oils – is the first step towards achieving better health. Here is a list of cooking oils and their principal type of fat content. Each has different health benefits.

Cooking oil

Saturated
coconut
palm
butter
lard
margarine

Polyunsaturated
safflower
sunflower
walnut
grapeseed
soya bean
pumpkin
corn
sesame

Monounsaturated
olive
almond
hazelnut
avocado
peanut (groundnut)
pistachio
rapeseed (canola)

Note: Most vegetable oils are a combination of mono- and polyunsaturates, so will contain both kinds of fats.

Unrefined tastes

You will notice that in referring to the type of oils we should be
eating I often use the all-important words 'natural' and 'unrefined'.

This is because it is not just the type of oil that matters, but the way it is processed is crucial too. The term 'natural' does not necessarily apply just to a substance itself, but also to the way it is produced. The chemical make-up of oil that ends up in a bottle on the supermarket shelf depends on the way it is refined. In olden times, oils were extracted by cold-pressing methods in which nuts and seeds underwent coarse grinding before being pressed to release the oil. This was (and still is) a time-consuming and costly exercise. It was also wasteful as it left much of the oil behind. It takes about 5kg of olives to make just 1 litre of cold-pressed olive oil, usually extracted from hard, unripe olives. In the 19th century, a screw-press method of extraction was invented that was more effective as it applied greater mechanical pressure to release the oils. Later still it was discovered that if the oil-laden nuts or seeds were heated up to a temperature of 100°C (212°F) before pressing, even more oil would be released. Although heated pressing is still used today to some extent, there are definite nutritional drawbacks. When polyunsaturated fatty acids are heated, it triggers oxidation, which means the fatty acid molecules combine with oxygen molecules at a much faster rate than normal. It is this oxidation that destroys some of the vital nutrients in oils, such as natural vitamin E and the essential fatty acids which are *essential* for achieving good health.

The main method of oil extraction used by cooking-oil manufacturers today is even more unappealing. Solvent extraction uses petroleum derivatives to dissolve the oils and make the whole extraction process faster and more effective. The main solvent used is hexane, a major component of petrol, which evaporates at relatively low temperatures.

Vegetable oil refining is a lengthy process. Here are just some of the stages:

○ Seeds are mechanically pressed at intense pressure and high temperatures up to 200°C (400°F).
○ Residual grounds are cooked and pressed again.
○ The remaining oilcake is mixed with solvent (such as

petroleum-based hexane). The solvent oil mixture is drained away from the residual cake and then heated to 150°C (300°F) and hexane removed by vacuum distillation.

○ The resulting dark, evil-smelling blend is de-gummed by re-heating and spraying with hot water. This removes valuable phospholipids, including lecithin.

○ Alkali refining using caustic soda destroys any remaining free fatty acids.

○ Natural pigments are removed by bleaching. This involves mixing the oil with earths or clays treated with acid to make them more absorbent. The pigments cling on to the earths and are filtered out.

○ Finally, the oil's natural flavours and aromas are removed by deodorisation. The oil is heated under conditions of high vacuum to 250°C (480°F) and pressurised steam is blown through to evaporate the compounds which give the oil its taste and smell. This also removes vitamin E, although traces of the solvent hexane may be left behind.

○ The devitalised end product may then receive a dose of synthetic vitamins to replace those lost during the refining process. This means that the oil can then be legally termed 'pure'!

By contrast, unrefined oils are mini health treatments in themselves and contain naturally occurring nutrients such as vitamins D, E and EFAs, all of which are highly beneficial to the body and skin whether taken internally or used topically on the skin. Unrefined oils tend to involve the single mechanical pressing of the seeds at temperatures, usually below 80°C (175°F). The oil is then filtered and bottled.

The only method of extraction that preserves the original goodness is cold-pressing. Any chef will also tell you that unrefined, cold-pressed oils are the tastiest, because refining drives away the volatile flavour compounds that give certain oils their unique flavour. Unfortunately, cold-pressed oils are the most inefficient to produce and are also the most expensive, which explains why virgin olive oil made from the first pressing of olives can cost even more than champagne. The most 'artisan' and expensive cooking oils tend to be the least refined and are likely to contain higher levels of natural vitamins than refined oils. However, always buy from a reputable company that has the resources to test for purity. Cold-pressed vegetable oils can contain high levels of fungal spores as well as occasional traces of undesirable metals, such as cadmium, lead and mercury. Buying from an established company with a reputation for quality may be the best route. When in doubt, ask your supplier.

Choosing a cooking oil

As the benefits of cold-pressed oils have become more widely known, so they have become increasingly available, but unfortunately there is no legislation to control the exact labelling of oils. An oil can state that it has been cold-pressed even if it has subsequently been subjected to heat-treating or further refined after the cold pressing. In addition, the crushing process may have been carried out with great force or speed that generates its own heat, technically making the oil warm pressed. Some honest oil producers have recognised this difficulty and describe their products as 'unrefined', which is probably the most accurate description. Other manufacturers are not so up-front, making it extremely difficult for us to know exactly what is in the bottle.

Another option is to choose from the wide selection of organically produced cooking oils available, as these are subject to more stringent production processes to qualify for organic certification. Organic growers meeting the required standards are awarded the various logos that appear on the bottle's label, e.g. the Soil Association in the UK, Ecocert in France and Demeter in Germany. The UK's Soil Association sets some of the highest standards in the world and is a good label to choose. When in doubt, here are a few helpful hints that can help you get the best buys:

○ Choose oils that are naturally darker in colour and have a nutty smell. This means the oil has not been bleached or deodorised.
○ Stick to single oils instead of those that say they are an

anonymous blend of several different varieties. With a pure oil, at least you know what you should be getting.

○ Choose oils that have been packaged to protect them from rancidity caused by exposure to the light. Look for dark-coloured glass bottles or metal tins.

○ Check the best-before date. Unrefined oils should keep for nine months due to their natural antioxidants. Seriously good oils, like fine wine, will also list the date when they were bottled.

○ All oils should be stored away from bright lights, so only buy from shops that have a rapid turnover and have not left them on the shelves for months on end.

○ As with wine, every time you take the top off an oil bottle, the contents come under attack from oxygen molecules, so choose smaller bottles and replace more frequently instead of buying in bulk. Always replace the cap after opening.

○ If you are planning a lengthy trip away from home or have surplus good-quality cooking oils to store, you can safely place bottles in the freezer for up to two years. Unlike water or alcohol, oil shrinks when frozen so glass bottles will not break.

When you have bought your oils, make sure to store them in a cool, dark place away from sunlight. Some natural clouding may occur (particularly in cold weather) and is a welcome sign that the oil has not been refined or excessively filtered. The fridge is one of the best places to keep oil and a few days of cold-storage will reveal more about the oil too. If it looks cloudy or develops sediment, don't panic – all this means is that the saturated portion of the oil has sunk to the bottom, a process that is encouraged by refrigeration. If you want to reduce your saturated fatty acid levels, simply leave this inch or so behind in the bottle. Unrefined vegetable oils that still have their nutrients will quickly lose them if stored at room temperature. Safflower oil loses more than half its vitamin E after three months and corn oil loses more than a third after six months. The exception to using cold storage is olive oil, which can solidify at low temperatures. However, olive oil is more resistant to damage by heat and light than polyunsaturated oils and can be more safely stored at room temperature.

Cooking with oils

Once you've bought your oil, the problems that occur when it is heated mean that you must carefully choose your cooking method too. Heating oil to a high temperature, say in a chip pan, destroys many of the healthy properties we want to preserve. When oil is heated above 100°C (212°F) it not only wipes out important nutrients, but also generates free radicals – destructive molecular fragments that have been implicated in multiple cell damage leading to all kinds of health scares, from heart disease to cancer and even premature skin ageing. However, Nature has an innate sense of balance and many vegetable oils are naturally enriched with vitamin E, a nutrient renowned for its extraordinary health-giving properties. Most important of these is its ability to seek out and neutralise free radicals, thereby minimising the amount of internal cell damage. But as vitamin E is also destroyed in the heating process, using oils at high temperatures not only creates free radicals but also destroys the ability to combat them. Peanut oil, for example, is a rich source of vitamin E, but frying it at high temperatures will reduce its vitamin E levels by one-third.

Among the least stable oils for cooking are sunflower, safflower and soya bean, all of which produce free radicals when heated. All vegetable oils that are rich in EFAs are destroyed to some extent by heating and the less they are damaged, the better they are for us. Vegetable oils are therefore generally best kept for use at low temperatures or for using cold in marinades and dressings. If you want the occasional fry-up, a little bit of butter is probably your best choice, followed by the solid tropical fats, such as palm or coconut. Other good choices for frying, according to the dietary oil expert Dr Udo Erasmus, are (in order of preference): high oleic sunflower and high oleic safflower oil (available from larger health food shops), peanut (groundnut) and olive oil. Dr Erasmus also suggests adding sulphur-rich garlic and onions to the pan when frying to help minimise free radical damage. But he does say that to obtain the very best of health, frying and deep-frying should be banned! If you do fry with a vegetable oil, only use the oil once and never re-heat. You don't need to use the most expensive varieties – an inexpensive blend of peanut and rapeseed is good to keep in the fridge for occasional use. The key is to avoid frying in temperatures that are too high and never to let the oil residues go brown (or worse still, turn black). This is an indication that the oil is producing potentially cancer-causing compounds.

However, not all experts agree. According to Dr Ray Rice, one of the UK's leading 'fat' specialists, olive oil is not only the best choice for frying but it can safely be used for deep-fat frying and re-used many times over. This is because it only contains 5–6 per cent linoleic acid and so is much more robust than other vegetable oils. When it comes to the issue of frying, the best option of all is to invest in a cast iron frying pan that will 'dry fry' foods such as eggs, onions and bacon.

BUTTER OR SPREAD?

You may have been surprised to read that butter may be one of the better choices for our health when it comes to baking and frying. This is because it is high in saturated fat, which, although not good for the body in excess, is usefully more stable at higher temperatures than the polyunsaturated fats. The changes that take place at high temperatures happen more rapidly in polyunsaturated fats – and unfortunately even faster in oils that are rich in healthy EFAs. Frying turns EFAs into toxic materials that can damage health, whereas the saturated fats in butter are only minimally damaged.

So, does this mean that butter beats sunflower spread when it comes to the question of what to spread on our bread? There is no easy answer to this and the butter vs. margarine/low-fat spread debate looks set to rage for many years to come. The question is constantly fought out by the marketing campaigns of both the dairy industry and the oil processors, each side producing compelling arguments. The processed spread business is certainly hugely profitable.

The spreads are cheap to make and a high profit margin means there is ample funding for biased advertising campaigns. About half of the entire sunflower oil crop is bought by the food industry for making margarine and low-fat spreads. There is so much confusion and controversy surrounding the health benefits of butter vs. spreads that it is worth dwelling awhile on the complex issues involved.

Although butter is relatively high in saturated fat, it is favoured by many for being a pure, natural product. Butter contains butyric acid and other short-chain fatty acids that are easy to digest. However, it is low in EFAs and high in fats that can interfere with the enzymes that help us utilise the beneficial EFAs, so an excess of butter is clearly not a good idea. Butter also contains cholesterol and, as already discussed, although this is not a villain in itself, an excess is not desirable. Another important point is that conventionally produced butter can contain pesticide residues stored in animal fat cells, as well as traces of hormone treatments, antibiotics and other bovine medications either routinely given to cattle or contained in their feed, though the risk of contamination from these can be reduced by buying organic butter. In addition, butter also contains small amounts of trans fatty acids (see opposite) that are produced by bacteria in a cow's stomach, but these are in much smaller amounts than in the processed spreads and are probably less harmful than those created by the hydrogenation processes involved in margarine manufacture. On the plus side, butter is stable at higher temperatures and can be safely used for baking and light frying. So, although butter has few direct health benefits, the use of organically produced butter is useful because it is easy to digest, is good for cooking and in small amounts it will not disrupt the delicate balance of EFAs in the body. Let's not forget that butter also tastes great!

Margarine was originally invented in France under Napoleon III, who was looking for a cheap source of fat for both the army and the poor. During the Second World War, it was further developed as an alternative to butter during food rationing and has remained a constant part of our diet ever since. Today, in contrast to butter, margarine and low-fat spreads are highly processed products made with complicated chemical wizardry. Since the discovery that, overall, polyunsaturates are better for us than saturates, many soft margarines based on sunflower oil have appeared on the market. If a soft spread makes any claim about polyunsaturates on the label it must satisfy strict food labelling laws. At least 45 per cent of its fat content must be poly-unsaturated and not more than 25 per cent can be saturated. While these sunflower spreads are a useful source of polyunsaturates, they have about the same number of calories as butter and should not be confused with low-fat 'diet' spreads. These are far lower in calories and consist of half fat and half water, but much of their fat is the satu-rated variety. So although low-fat spreads contain fewer calories, the fat content tends to be less desirable for overall health.

Although margarine and soft spreads contain plenty of EFAs, their partial hydrogenation destroys many of their health-giving proper-ties. These processed spreads also contain significant amounts of arti-ficially created trans fatty acids. (For more information on trans fats see p.9.) In the long term, this means that eating too many trans fats can actually lead to a lack of important essential fatty acids.

Trans fatty acids have been linked to many serious diseases, including heart disease and cancer. As they also block the positive action of the beneficial fats that we get from our food their action in our bodies is a double negative. Most trans fats come from partially hydrogenated vegetable oils and are found in many processed foods (often not revealed on the label) as well as margarine and processed spreads. The good news is that technology has improved in the 'spreadable fats' industry in recent years and it is now much easier to buy spreads that contain no trans fats, no cholesterol, no hydro-genated fats and plenty of beneficial EFAs. These new spreads tend to be made in a similar way to mayonnaise, although they may contain additives such as salt, preservatives and artificial flavourings. If you do buy one of these spreads, make sure that it's rich in vitamin E to help protect the integrity of the vegetable oils it contains.

Other problems with spreads relate to the lack of information revealed on their labels. Although hydrogenated fats have largely been removed, they are often replaced with palm or coconut oils, both short-chain saturated fats. Some researchers argue that these tropical fats may even be worse for us than hydrogenated poly-unsaturates. Unfortunately, the labelling of these spreads is a grey area and the makers don't have to specify whether they are using palm, coconut or (healthier) rapeseed oils. These may all come under the vague term of 'vegetable oils'. Unless a pack fully identifies precisely what oils it contains, it is probably best not to buy it.

My own personal preference in the butter *vs.* spread debate is to use small amounts of pure, organic butter for cooking and for its delicious taste. If I need something that spreads more easily from the fridge, I make my own 'spread' by blending roughly equal quantities of softened butter with unrefined olive oil in a food mixer and storing it in a tub in the fridge.

LECITHIN

When choosing which oils to use for eating and general cooking, the word 'lecithin' frequently crops up on food labels. Lecithin is a phospholipid – a substance that helps our body deal with oils and fats more effectively. There are many different phospholipids, but lecithin is the most widely known and probably the most important. Lecithin contains choline, a chemical needed for healthy brain and nerve function. It is also vitally important to help our liver to process the many fats in our diet properly. As the liver is involved in almost all serious diseases (a poor liver function is frequently a forerunner of cancer) it makes sense to supply the liver with enough lecithin to help it work properly. Lecithin has been described as an 'edible detergent' as it helps to keep cholesterol soluble, dissolving gall and kidney stones by breaking down the fatty deposits that can cause them. Lecithin is also an important part of bile, a liquid that we need to break down our fatty foods into more digestible droplets of emulsified oils.

We often obtain lecithin in food via the foods that animals eat before us – for example, if hens are fed with lecithin-rich feed, we eat eggs containing lecithin. Meat from animals fed with good-quality foodstuffs will also be naturally higher in lecithin than those fed with on a poor diet. This is yet another argument in favour of choosing to eat only organically reared produce, as this tends to be produced with greater attention to the detail of an animal's diet.

NUT OIL ALLERGIES

About one in every 100 people in the UK are sensitive to peanuts and the figures are rising, especially among the young. This is a serious problem for many families and one that can result in the severe allergic reaction, anaphylactic shock, which can be fatal. However, the proteins that cause this extreme allergic reaction are totally removed when peanut oil is refined. This has led to declarations that refined peanut oil is completely safe for those with nut allergies – to such an extent that it may not even be identified on a food label that simply states 'vegetable' oil. The UK Department of Health Committee on Toxicity of Chemicals in Food, Consumer Products and the Environment consider that 'the use of refined oil in food and medical products is without risk to sensitive individuals. Refined peanut oil is therefore not included in the category 'peanut products''. Although refined peanut oil (also known as groundnut oil) is safe to consume, some studies are less sure that it should be applied to the skin, especially if the skin is broken or inflamed (for example, in the case of weeping eczema). Researchers have found that using peanut oil on the skin of young children may be one of the triggers that can cause an allergic reaction, although there have been no reported effects from the general use of toiletries containing peanut oils. This is probably because the peanut oil used by the cosmetics industry is also highly refined. If you have a history of nut allergies in the family it would be advisable in this instance either to avoid nut oils altogether, or to choose brands that have been refined. Cold-pressed, artisan hazelnut, sesame and walnut oils may look tempting, but could potentially trigger an allergic reaction.

According to the UK Institute of Food Science and Technology there are over 170 foods documented in scientific literature as causing allergic reactions. Of these, the 'big eight' are (in order) milk, eggs, soya, wheat, peanuts, shellfish, fruits and tree nuts, which between them account for most food allergies. The 'second eight' are (in order) sesame seeds, sunflower seeds, poppy seed, molluscs, beans (other than green beans), peas and lentils. The Institute states that 'fully refined peanut oils and tree nut oils do not cause allergic reactions in sensitive subjects, but unrefined oils do'. In addition, the British Retail Consortium produces a 'nut' classification list to illustrate to food manufacturers which nuts are known to cause anaphylactic shock reactions, for the purpose of food labelling. This list includes almond, Brazil, cashew, chestnut, hazel, macadamia, peanut, pecan, pistachio and walnut.

A–Z guide to cooking oils

The following alphabetical guide describes common cooking oils in detail. Always choose the unrefined versions, so long as you are not allergic to the foods from which they are extracted.

CORN OIL (*Zea mays*)

Background: Corn or maize oil is high in polyunsaturates (57 per cent on average) and is one of the cheapest, most commonly used oils for cooking. Corn oil comes from the corn-on-the-cob plant and is extracted from the sweetcorn kernels.

Science: Most corn oil comes from the USA and southern France where it is usually heavily refined for blended cooking oils. However, it is possible to find pure, unrefined versions in health food shops and larger supermarkets. Unrefined corn oil contains useful levels of the natural antioxidant vitamin E (about 66mg per 100g).

When I wrote the first edition of *Vital Oils* in 1990, genetic modification of foods had not even been mentioned. Since then, a huge outcry has occurred with the development of some genetically engineered crops. Maize, along with the soya bean, is one of the few foods currently being widely genetically engineered. Almost all the maize and soya products we eat today will have been genetically tampered with. The only way to make sure that you are eating foods that are GM-free is to make sure the label says so. Blended cooking oils are most likely to contain genetically engineered ingredients such as maize and soya bean.

Benefits and uses: Being a polyunsaturated oil, corn oil is a good source of the omega-6 essential fatty acids. Corn oil deteriorates when heated to high temperatures, so is best kept for recipes that use it cold or warm, such as sauces. Some cooks consider corn oil to be too heavy to use in salad dressings. Also, as a polyunsaturated oil, it needs protecting from heat, light and exposure to the air. It is best bought in small quantities so you use it up faster and should be stored in the fridge. Inexpensive dressings can be made using corn oil as a base with small quantities of the more expensive nut oils added for flavour.

GRAPESEED OIL (*Vitis vinifera*)

Background: Grapeseed oil comes from grape pips and, not surprisingly, most of the oil we import comes from the wine-growing regions of France. Although the grapevine has been around for thousands of years, commercial oil extraction from the squashed pips is a fairly new process. The pips are washed, dried, ground and pressed with the aid of heat and, mostly, further refined.

Science: Grapeseed oil has one of the highest polyunsaturated fatty acid contents, second only to safflower. Unrefined grapeseed oil has a very unpleasant smell and so is not generally available. Refined grapeseed oil is light and taste-free and so is a useful neutral base for salad dressings to which more nutritious oils are added. Because it has a fine texture and no smell, refined grapeseed oil is also useful as a massage oil. It has a high smoke point, which means that it can be heated to higher temperatures before giving off a bluish-coloured smoke. When an oil starts to smoke it is a sign that it has started to break down and should be thrown away – never re-heated!

Benefits and uses: Grape pips can be distilled to produce grapeseed extract. This expensive skincare ingredient is one of the richest natural sources of antioxidants and can be used in formulations to help prevent free radical skin damage.

GROUNDNUT OIL (*Arachis hypogaea*)

Background: Groundnut oil, or peanut oil, comes from peanut kernels. The peanut plant belongs to the same legume family as the soya bean. It is a hardy annual that thrives on a light soil and subtropical climate, is fast-growing and will produce its first crop of peanuts just four months after planting. The peanut plant is mainly cultivated in developing countries as it can be harvested by hand. It is an important crop in Nigeria and other parts of West Africa, China, South America and India.

Science: Technically, the kernels are not nuts at all but seed pods that develop underground. Groundnut oil is usually highly refined and also loses many of its healthy attributes in processing. Unrefined groundnut oil is a useful source of vitamin E (around 21mg per 100ml). It is monounsaturated (about 48 per cent of its content) but also has a good level of polyunsaturated fatty acids (about 28 per cent). As with rapeseed and soyabean oils, groundnut oil has a high smoke point so is often recommended for shallow-frying.

Benefits and uses: Peanuts in their raw state are highly nutritious and consist of about 45 per cent oil, 30 per cent protein and valuable quantities of iron, vitamin B (niacin) and vitamin E. Peanuts are best eaten straight from their shells as much of their nutritional benefit is lost when processed as 'dry-roasted' snacks.

HAZELNUT OIL (*Corylus avellana*)

Background: Although one of the newer vegetable oils to appear in the supermarket, hazelnut oil is thought to have first been extracted during the Bronze Age. Hazelnuts, also known as cobnuts or filberts, originate from a tall shrub that grows wild throughout Europe. The best-quality hazelnut oils are hand-produced and come from France, where gourmet cooks praise it for its sweet, smooth flavour. However, it is one of the more expensive oils, so is best used in small amounts to flavour salad dressings and sauces.

Science: Hazelnuts are a nutritious food, being amongst the lowest in fat of the nuts and containing useful levels of vitamin E. Hazelnut oil is most commonly warm-pressed from the small nut kernels. After pressing, the hazelnut oil is left to settle in vats, where it takes about a week for the sediment to separate and sink to the bottom. On average, 2.5kg of hazelnuts will yield about 1 litre of oil.

Benefits and uses: Hazelnut oil is monounsaturated and contains a high level of oleic acid (about 80 per cent), so it can be gently heated without damaging its chemical structure. It also contains useful levels of omega-6 linoleic acid (up to 20 per cent). Hazelnut oil is wonderful for baking and a few drops added to nutty cake and biscuit mixtures give a deliciously subtle taste. It will keep for up to a year while sealed. Once opened, store in a cool, dark place or in the fridge.

OLIVE OIL (*Olea europea*)

Background: Olive oil is the king of oils and has legendary health and beauty properties. Since the early days of mankind, the olive tree has been a powerful symbol of strength, peace and fertility. The Ancient Egyptians were amongst the first to use olive oil, regarding it as a gift from their great goddess, Isis. Large casks of olive oil were entombed alongside the pharaohs and garlands of olive branches were found crowning the head of Tutankhamun.

The Ancient Greeks also valued olive oil, believing it to be a gift from the goddess Athena, while the Hebrews have valued the olive tree since the time of Adam. The Bible contains some of the earliest references to the olive – in the Book of Exodus, Moses is told how to make an anointing oil from spiced olives, and in the story of the Great Flood Noah's dove is described returning to the ark clutching an olive branch in its beak. Early civilisations used olive oil as a form of currency and it provided fuel for their lamps as well as being a food and medicine. The Greek poet Homer referred to olive oil as liquid gold and the fathers of medicine, Hippocrates and Galen, prescribed it for sunburn. Pedacius Dioscorides, who wrote one of the first manuscripts on herbal medicine during the first century AD, also used olive oil to treat stomach disorders.

Science: Most olive oil now comes from Spain, Italy, Greece and southern France, where the plentiful Mediterranean sunshine, moderate rain and enriched soil suits the cultivated olive tree. Each tree produces 10–20kg of olives a year and the oil is usually pressed in local olive mills located near the groves. Spain is the world's leading olive grower and has some 200 million trees producing between

450,000 and 750,000 metric tons of olive oil every year. The olives grown for pressing are soft and squashy, unlike the firmer varieties grown for the table. There are about 60 different oil-bearing varieties, all of which are green at first and turn black as they ripen. Although it takes up to ten years before an olive tree bears its first fruit, it is long-lived and can flourish for 600 years or more.

There are four main olive oil regions in Spain and each produces an oil that differs in flavour and appearance from the rest. Because their flavours are so diverse, the oils from these areas are awarded Labels of Origin which state where the olives were grown and whether the oil is the result of an early harvest (slightly bitter) or a late harvest (paler and sweeter). Olive oil varies in taste and colour from year to year depending on the variety of olives used and the time of harvesting. As with fine wines, the taste also depends largely on the climate and growing conditions, but, unlike vintage claret, olive oil doesn't improve with age. Olive oil labels can be read in the same way as wine labels to reveal the quality and taste of their contents. The best Spanish oils come from Borjas Blancas, Siurana, Baena and Sierra de Segura. All four areas produce the best quality extra virgin olive oils, classified as having less than 1 per cent acidity.

Compared to other nut and seed oils, olive oil is one of the simplest to process. It was originally extracted by crushing olives in hessian bags suspended in barrels of water. When the oil floated to the top of the barrels it was skimmed off and bottled. Nowadays most olive oil is extracted by cold-pressing, and it is still the easiest type of oil to find in its raw, unrefined state. Virgin oil is classified as the unrefined juice of the fruit with an acidity level of less than 2 per cent. Extra virgin olive oil has an acidity level of less than 1 per cent and is the best – and most expensive – type you can buy. Bottles labelled 'pure' olive oil are not as unadulterated as their name implies and contain a blend of both refined and virgin olive oils. Supermarket own-labels and well-known brands may be extracted using a combination of heat and solvents, and are mixed to a standard recipe so they taste the same every time.

The most pungent, full-flavoured olive oils are dark green in colour and their powerful aromas are best suited for sparing use in dressings and sauces. Olive oil is one of the longest-lasting oils as it forms fewer of the degenerating peroxides that cause rancidity when exposed to heat or daylight. Unlike some cooking oils, it produces fewer of the dangerous substances, peroxides and aldehydes, that have toxic effects in the body. So for the occasional fry-up, olive oil is the best type of oil to choose, as its chemical structure remains the most stable at high temperatures. In cooking terms, at least, olive oil probably has the fewest number of negative factors and the greatest number of health-giving properties.

Benefits and uses: The link between olive oil and heart disease was first discovered by scientists at the University of Minnesota who undertook an extensive study into the worldwide numbers of deaths from heart disease. They discovered that the death rates were lowest amongst those whose main source of dietary fat was olive oil. One of the lowest incidences of heart disease is in Crete where the oil flows like wine and the native population receives up to half its calorific intake from olive oil alone. Not only do they cook exclusively with the stuff, the Cretans also knock back a glass or two as a preprandial aperitif. The Italians are also great consumers of olive oil and their incidence of heart disease is correspondingly low. The effects of olive oil on the system are certainly impressive and just two-thirds of a tablespoonful taken every day has been shown to lower blood pressure. Some doctors in Milan actually prescribe a daily dose of 60–75ml (4–5 tablespoonfuls) of olive oil to patients suffering from heart disease and thrombosis.

The reason olive oil has such a potent effect within the body lies in its chemical composition. Olive oil is dominated by monounsaturated fatty acids (about 70 per cent of its overall content) which alter the overall cholesterol balance in the bloodstream in a more beneficial way than polyunsaturated vegetable oils. This is because olive oil lowers total cholesterol levels while preserving the 'good' HDL type of cholesterol. This action preserves the important protective ratios of HDLs to LDLs, unlike polyunsaturated fats, which knock out both good and bad forms of cholesterol. Olive oil is now widely regarded as being as effective at combating high cholesterol levels as a low-fat diet, although too much saturated fat from meat and dairy products will block its health-giving action.

In addition to monounsaturated fatty acids, olive oil also contains over 1000 active chemical compounds, many of which are currently under investigation. One chemical called cycloarthanol seems to play a particularly important part in preventing the absorption of excess cholesterol in the body. Olive oil has also been found to have a similar ratio of EFAs as human breast milk and is good to use when preparing foods for small children. It is also a useful source of vitamin E (around 5mg per 100ml) which helps to protect the body from harmful free radical cell damage. Other benefits from olive oil include anti-coagulating agents that thin the blood, thus reducing the risk of blood clotting, and an ability to strengthen the delicate membranes surrounding the cells, making them less susceptible to free radical damage. Olive oil has traditionally been used for stomach disorders and we now know that it stimulates bile production and will encourage the gall bladder to contract, reducing the risk of gallstones. It also promotes pancreatic secretions and may even help protect against stomach ulcers.

RAPESEED OIL (*Brassica napus*)

Background: The first rapeseed crop in England was recorded as far back as 1381 and today it has become an important ingredient in commercially processed foods. The rape plant belongs to the cabbage family and grows to 1.5–1.8 metres (5–6 feet) high with vivid yellow flowers. Fields of these intense yellow flowers appears from May onwards and have become a familiar (and sometimes controversial) landmark in the British countryside. Rape is a favourite crop with British farmers because it forms humus, which enriches soil and helps to keep the ground healthy. It also gives the soil a much-needed break from growing wheat and is useful for farming crop rotation. Another reason for its popularity is the large EC farming subsidies for growing high-protein seed oil crops. Rape grows well all over Britain, but especially in Scotland as it favours a heavy soil and long summer days. Because of its unfortunate name, some prefer to call rape 'cole' and have renamed rapeseed coleseed. The Canadians have gone one step further and renamed their rapeseed oil 'Canola' oil and this name has been registered as a national brand trademark.

Science: Rape is certainly a versatile crop. The seeds contain 35–40 per cent pure oil, and the young leaves can also be served as a vegetable. The oil is used for commercial and domestic cooking, and also as an industrial lubricant. The French have also found a way of turning rapeseed oil into a less polluting form of diesel fuel. Both the plant and seedcake left over from the oil-refining process are popular cattle feeds, so very little of the plant is wasted.

Benefits and uses: Rapeseed oil has the highest percentage of unsaturated fats of any vegetable oil. Just over half of these are monounsaturated, with most of the rest being polyunsaturated. It is a light, versatile oil with no flavour that is a useful culinary staple. It can be flavoured with a few drops of the more expensive nut oils to make it more interesting in recipes. Rapeseed oil must be protected from light and heat to delay rancidity and is best stored in the fridge. A major nutritional aspect of rapeseed oil is that it has a favourable ratio of omega-6:omega-3 fats. The type of rapeseed oil in use in the UK has about 23 per cent of its fatty acids in the form of the omega-6 linoleic acid and about 11 per cent as omega-3 alpha-linolenic acid, which gives it an unusually good omega-6:omega-3 ratio of 2:1.

SAFFLOWER OIL (*Carthamus tinctorius*)

Background: The safflower belongs to the thistle family and originates from India. It grows up to 1.5 metres high and was originally cultivated for its reddish flowers which were used to dye cloth vibrant shades or orange and pink. The bitter safflower fruit was also used as a red vegetable dye which was favoured by the Ancient Egyptians for dyeing the cotton swaddling used for mummification. The safflower is now grown worldwide for the oil that can be extracted from its crop of tiny seeds. It is widely used in industry as a drying oil for paints, but is increasingly appreciated for its benefits in cooking and food-use too.

Science: Because safflower is cheap and easy to grow, it has become increasingly popular as a low-saturate cooking oil. High in polyunsaturates, unrefined safflower oil is rich in the omega-6 group of essential fatty acids. It has an extraordinarily high content of linoleic acid (up to 78 per cent) and up to 15 per cent oleic acid. However, because it is so high in polyunsaturates it is also very unstable and quickly breaks down when heated. Unrefined safflower oil is also a good source of vitamin E (49mg per 100ml). The unrefined oil has a rich, golden colour and it is possible to find organically grown versions.

Benefits and uses: Safflower oil has an attractive, nutty taste and is excellent in salad dressings. However, as it is one of the least stable oils at high temperatures it should not be used for frying. If you do want to fry with safflower oil, choose one that states it has been developed to create a high oleic acid content, as this will be more stable at high temperatures. There are several other, better options for frying, including olive or rapeseed oil. Normal safflower oil is one of the most difficult vegetable oils to keep fresh and should always be stored in the fridge.

SESAME OIL (*Sesamum indicum*)

Background: Sesame oil was used in British cooking as far back as Roman times and is one of the oldest seed oils known to mankind. Evidence indicates Ethiopia as the centre of its original cultivation and a 4000-year-old drawing on an Egyptian tomb depicts a baker adding sesame seeds to the dough. The sesame plant grows to about three metres high and resembles garden mint. Its sweet-smelling funnel-shaped flowers are a vivid shade of pink and are highly prized by the perfume industry. The sesame plant bears small nuts, each covered with hooks to snag the coats of grazing animals and ensure seed dispersal. The seeds are contained in four tiny compartments within the nut. Sesame oil is used in the manufacture of some margarines and in its unrefined state is one of the most versatile cooking oils.

Science: Being both a mono- and polyunsaturated oil, it can be heated to higher temperatures than high polyunsaturated oils with less risk of forming toxic elements. Its EFA content is roughly balanced between mono- and polyunsaturated fatty acids. Sesame oil may also be heated and sold as toasted sesame oil, although this process does destroy much of its nutrients. This has a wonderfully pungent flavour and just a few drops add zest to salad dressings and marinades.

Benefits and uses: Sesame seeds themselves are a tasty source of iron, calcium and protein and can be crushed to make the oily paste tahini. They are also used to make the Greek sweetmeat, halva, a nutritious form of fudge. Due to its high content of natural antioxidants (sesamol), sesame oil is a relatively stable vegetable oil. Both types of sesame oil should be stored in a cool, dry place.

SOYA BEAN OIL (*Glycine max*)

Background: Soya bean oil comes from the soya plant, which belongs to the pea or legume family. It is a relative newcomer to the cooking oil market, although it has a long and illustrious culinary history. Soya beans can be traced back 5000 years to their first recorded cultivation in Mainland China, where they are still grown today, as well as in Japan, the USA and Brazil. There are over 1000 different varieties of the soya plant, ranging from small busy shrubs to tall, leafy plants. The plants are unusual in that they must spend a certain length of time in complete darkness in order to flower and germinate. For this reason, soya beans are impossible to grow in places of northern latitudes (such as Britain) that have relatively short summer nights.

Science: The oil is extracted from smooth egg-shaped beans that are usually yellow but may be black or green in colour. Their oil content is low (13–20 per cent) and, for reasons of economy, are invariably extracted with solvents. Although soya bean oil is one of our cheapest cooking oils, it is almost impossible to find it in an unrefined state. When unrefined, soya bean oil is our second-best source of vitamin E (87mg per 100ml) after wheatgerm oil and contains more lecithin than any other vegetable oil. It also contains all 22 of the health-giving amino acids, along with beta-carotene and the B complex vitamins – so the unrefined version is worth searching for! Soya bean oil has a high level of polyunsaturates (around 56 per cent) and so produces toxic elements when heated at high temperatures.

Benefits and uses: The reasons why soya bean oil is so nutritious stem from the intriguing soya bean itself which deserves a special mention. Soya beans must be the world's most nutritious and versatile source of food, and in China they are nicknamed 'meat without bones'. Not only do they have a useful oil content, but they are also one of the very best sources of vegetable protein. Soya beans are widely used in vegetarian, vegan and macrobiotic cookery and can be processed to create several different types of food, such as tofu, tempeh and soya milk and cream.

SUNFLOWER OIL (*Helianthus anuus*)

Background: The sunflower first appeared in Mexico and Peru and its botanical name comes from the Greek word *helios*, meaning 'sun' and *anthos*, meaning 'flower'. In France, the plant is called *tournesol* and in Italy *girasole*, both of which mean 'turn towards the sun' but, although the flowers do all grow facing the same way, they do not actually turn to follow the sun. Sunflowers can grow to five metres (15 feet) high and have a large circular seed head surrounded by soft yellow petals that resemble the sun's rays. They were an important plant to the Aztecs who worshipped the sun and forged replicas of the flower in gold to line their temple walls. Sunflowers are extremely fast-growing and will thrive on poor soil provided they get several hours of full sunshine. The roots of the sunflower plant are highly efficient at sucking water out of the soil and sunflowers are often planted in areas that require drainage – large areas of the Netherlands are planted with them. It is a versatile plant and every part of it can be used. The petals can be steeped in water to make a yellow hair dye, the woody stalks are used in papermaking and the oil is extracted from the seeds. The principal sunflower-oil-producing countries are Russia, Romania, Hungary, Argentina, France, Australia and South Africa.

Science: Light and slightly sweet, sunflower oil is extracted from the sunflower seeds as soon as they have fully ripened and turned black. The seeds contain about 40 per cent oil and are also delicious eaten raw. They make a nourishing snack and are a good source of calcium, protein, vitamins B1, B6, zinc and potassium.

Benefits and uses: Sunflower seeds can be sprouted on damp blotting paper and make a nutritious ingredient for salads. Sunflower oil is very high in polyunsaturates and when unrefined contains useful amounts of omega-6 essential fatty acids. The natural oil also contains relatively high levels of vitamin E (27mg per 100ml). Sunflower oil is used extensively in blended cooking oils, although unfortunately most of these are highly processed and low in nutrients. However, the unrefined versions are inexpensive and easily available from health food stores. Sunflower oil is best used cold or at low temperatures as it is very high in polyunsaturates (around 63 per cent) and so breaks down and produces toxic elements when heated to high temperatures. It should also be stored in the fridge.

WALNUT OIL (*Juglans regia*)

Background: Walnut oil is a relative newcomer to Britain, but features strongly in even quite basic French cooking. Traditionally, French chefs use a few drops to fry eggs and it is a good addition to salad dressings. Although the USA is the largest producer of walnuts, followed by China and Turkey, most of our walnut oil comes from France and the main areas of production are around Perigord, the Dordogne and the Loire.

Science: Oil extraction is a time-consuming process, as the shells often have to be removed by hand, using a small mallet on a stone base, taking care not to break the kernel. The kernels are then ground using a millstone and warm-pressed to release the oil. After pressing, the topaz-coloured oil is filtered through cotton cloth or paper before bottling. It takes about 2kg of walnuts to produce 1 litre of walnut oil. The oil is easy to find in its natural, unrefined state and is stocked in an increasing number of supermarkets. You will sometimes find it with its French label, Huile de Noix or Huile de Noix Extra (a slightly stronger flavour). Walnut oil is polyunsaturated, with both omega-6 and omega-3 EFAs present, and also contains low levels of GLA. It is at its best when used cold in dressings and sauces.

Benefits and uses: Although it is more expensive than other oils, a few drops go a long way and it makes a tasty addition to many recipes.

As an example, try adding a few drops to walnut cakes or biscuits to enhance the flavour. Unopened walnut oil will keep for up to a year if stored away from the light, but once open it is best kept in the fridge.

Easy ways to add vital oils to your diet

I suggest adding about 15ml (1 tablespoonful) of pure, plain, uncooked plant oil to foods each day for maximum health benefits. This can be in the form of salad dressings or simply added to everyday foods to enrich their nutritional benefit. Adding just this small quantity daily will help to ensure that we receive a good daily supply of the important essential fatty acids needed to protect us against disease, guard our mental health and promote stronger, smoother skin. Don't worry about the calories as each tablespoonful only contains about 160 Kcals, which is roughly equivalent to a handful of salted peanuts or a couple of biscuits – but, of course, a lot better for us. Fish oils are also vitally important and we should aim to eat 400–500mg a day of the omega-3, long-chain essential fatty acids, although this will need to be increased to achieve a therapeutic effect for any specific skin conditions and other ailments. Vegetarians who can't eat any fish would be advised to reduce their overall intake of linoleic acid from vegetable oils such as sunflower oil and increase the amount of alpha-linolenic acid they receive from flax oil. Vegetarians who eat marine algae will also benefit from choosing fortified foods such as Vitaquell spread, which is enriched with omega-3 essential fats from algae. Here are some ideas on how to add *vital oils* into your day-to-day diet:

BREAKFAST
Stir a little oil into low-fat yogurt. Mix a spoonful into muesli or porridge.

MILK AND FRUIT SMOOTHIES
Simply whizz up your favourite ingredients in a liquidiser. Use semi-skimmed milk, soya milk or fruit juice with extra low-fat yogurt or soya yogurt as a base, then add some fresh fruit such as a banana,

peach or a handful of strawberries. Finish with 15–30ml (1–2 table-spoonfuls) of oil per person. Walnut or rapeseed are good to try.

DIPS

Make quick and easy crudité dips based on low-fat soft cheese, fromage frais, Quark or yogurt. Add a little flavouring, choosing from French mustard, tomato purée, Worcestershire sauce, Tabasco, lemon juice and zest, fresh garlic, grated cucumber or freshly chopped herbs. Finish with 15ml (1 tablespoonful) of oil. Hazelnut or walnut gives an excellent flavour. Serve with thin slices of crisp raw vegetables.

SPREADS

Mix 30ml (2 tablespoonfuls) of Quark, low-fat soft cheese or cottage cheese with 1 finely chopped spring onion, 1 teaspoonful each of olive, sunflower (or safflower or rapeseed) and pumpkin oil. Season with celery salt and cayenne pepper to taste. Spread onto bread, rice cakes or crackers. Alternatively, add a spoonful or crushed olive paste, to taste, for a delicious alternative to tapenade.

STIR-FRIES AND STEAMED VEGETABLES

Oils are most potent when unheated so stir-fry with the minimum quantity of oil, then just before serving toss in an extra 15ml (1 table-spoonful) to glaze the vegetables. You can also add oils in this way to steamed vegetables to give them an appetising, glossy shine.

YOGURT, FRUIT AND NUT DESSERTS

Make unusual and delicious desserts based on live low-fat yogurt, goat's milk, sheep's milk or soya yogurt. Add chopped or liquidised fresh fruit, finely chopped or ground almonds or hazelnuts plus 15ml (1 tablespoonful) of oil per person. Choose from unrefined corn, sunflower, sesame or safflower oils.

HERB-FLAVOURED OILS

Herbs infuse well in vegetable oils to make delicious dressings and useful additions to recipes. Crushed garlic cloves make a wonderful addition to olive oil – use to lightly fry chops, steak and vegetables or for making quick and easy garlic bread. Basil, fennel (seeds and leaves), rosemary and marjoram also infuse well in olive, sunflower and hazelnut oil. An infusion made with dried chilli peppers will pep-up pizza and sausages. Home-made herbal oils must be kept cool (ideally refrigerated) and used within a few days. It is extremely rare, but fatalities have occurred from the poison botulism breeding in warm herb oils kept for long periods.

CANNED FISH

Few things beat opening a tin of tuna for convenience. Unfortunately, tuna is not high in valuable fish oils unless it is fresh or frozen. Buy tuna packed in brine and add a few drops of walnut or rapeseed oil to make it tastier – and healthier. Tinned mackerel fillets packed in tomato or mustard sauces also make a useful oily fish lunch, supper or snack.

Losing weight with vital oils

The rapid promotion of low-fat, no-fat diets in recent years has led us to be fearful of the fats and oils in our foods. But eating the right kinds of oils and fats actually helps the body to burn energy faster and can boost the metabolism, leading to faster weight loss. Oils are relatively high-calorie, energy-giving foods, so how can they help us slim? The answer is to revise the type of oils we eat and to cut out the over-refined and saturated kind that overload the body and clog up the system. Avoid all processed, damaged and hydrogenated fats (get into the habit of avid label reading in the supermarket) and focus instead on the energy-giving properties of the pure, natural *vital oils* mentioned throughout this book. Oil supplements are also a very useful way of increasing our daily oil intake and are remarkably low in calories. The average oil capsule, such as evening primrose oil or fish oil, contains just 3 Kcal (12.5 kJ) each. There are, in addition, many other important benefits to be gained from including a few drops of vital oils in our daily diet, including renewed energy levels, improvements to overall inner good health and outer radiance.

The first piece of positive action is to go through your shopping list and strike off the saturated fats. These block the actions of the cold-pressed vegetable and nut oils, and have no place in a health and beauty weight-loss plan. Definite results will be seen by avoiding cream, lard and suet and by reducing red meats and dairy products such as full-fat milk and cheese. Hardened margarine is high in saturated fats so should be avoided. Although polyunsaturated spreads are made with healthier oils, their structure may also have been changed by hydrogenation. As hydrogenation destroys an oil's health benefits, always choose unhydrogenated, softer spreads that boast a low trans fat content. As with any successful weight-loss plan, the emphasis must be on fresh, natural produce with plenty of fruit and vegetables, whole grains, beans, nuts and seeds, with some chicken or similarly lean meat for protein. A regular intake of fish oils is also highly beneficial, so choose recipes using oily fish such as mackerel, kippers, pilchards, trout, salmon, tuna, herring, sardines and anchovy.

Other useful sources of natural *vital oils* include lean meats, such as beef, chicken, venison and lamb (avoid processed pies, sausages etc.), nuts (especially walnuts and almonds) and vegetable oils such as rapeseed, walnut and soya oil. For good health, the British government advises eating one to two portions of oil-rich fish each week, which gives us around 2–3g of the omega-3 fish fats.

CLA FOR FASTER WEIGHT LOSS

Early research into one particular EFA is showing promise for help with speeding up weight loss. Conjugated Linoleic Acid (CLA) is a close relative of linoleic acid and is found naturally in many foods, such as beef and dairy products as when cattle are fed on grasses they convert some of its linoleic acid into CLA. However, with more intensively reared cows being fed on dried factory fodder, less CLA is ending up in our foods (yet another argument to support traditional or organic beef and dairy farming). In the late 1990s, clinical studies by researchers at the University of Wisconsin, amongst others in the USA, showed that CLA helps the body to maintain low body fat while supporting the development of lean muscle. More recent trials show that taking supplements of CLA may help to improve the ratio of body fat to lean muscle tissue (i.e make us look thinner, if not actually weigh less). In addition, CLA may have useful benefits in helping to support the immune system, glucose balance and bone density. Some nutritionists have suggested that CLA may help to normalise blood sugar metabolism, making it a potentially useful supplement for diabetics as well as those seeking to process foods more effectively. In addition, researchers in Finland have found that women with higher intakes of dairy products have a lower risk of breast cancer. This finding has been supported by a further study showing that those with higher levels of CLA in their blood may have a lower risk of developing breast cancer.

So, should we just be eating more steak and cheese to obtain our CLA supplies? Well, we could, but we'd need around 3kg of meat and 50 slices of cheese to get the same amount of CLA that is found in most food supplements. These tend to be made from sunflower oil, so are suitable for vegetarians or vegans who may be lacking in CLA and the usual recommended daily dose is three 1000mg capsules a day. As with all dietary supplements, there is no magic pill to melt away excess fat, however seductive some of the slimming industry claims might be (especially on the Internet, where the more outlandish claims are not regulated). It does seem, though, that CLA shows promise with helping to convert excess flab into leaner muscle mass. This is especially true if you can combine it with a sensible eating plan that contains only few processed, damaged fats from fast food and confectionery. You are likely to lose body fat when taking CLA, especially if you combine it with a modest increase in exercise. However, as lean muscle is heavier and more compact than fat, you may find that you actually weigh a little bit more – even if it's easier to fasten your waistband.

HELPFUL HINTS FOR SUCCESSFUL WEIGHT LOSS
○ There is no secret to successful weight-loss, but the *vital oils* can certainly play a helpful part in the process. Consider adding a food supplement that includes the EFAs from GLA, EPA and DHA as well as possible CLA for maximum benefit.

○ Cut down on stimulants such as tea, coffee and cola drinks that can disrupt the metabolism. Substitute with fresh fruit and vegetable juices (diluted with filtered water or low-salt mineral water).

○ Fruit and herb teas plus plenty of pure water (at least six glasses daily) will also speed the elimination of toxins and help to make you feel full.

○ Use lower fat skimmed or semi-skimmed milk. The taste is similar and yet the calorie content is much less.

○ Beware of high-fat dressings and mayonnaise and only use low-fat versions in moderation.

○ If you get hunger pangs between meals, snack on fibrous fruits such as apples, pears, oranges and grapes. These will cleanse and refresh the palate as well as stave off hunger attacks.

A word on weight reduction: A slow, steady weight loss is the best way to lose extra pounds and keep them off permanently. Rather than crash-dieting, it's worth incorporating a few drops of *vital oils* in your diet every day and for this habit to become a way of life. Remember, the food we eat not only gives us the energy to work, exercise and sleep well, but it also determines the quality of our skin, hair, blood, bones, muscles – in fact every possible part of us. It also helps to ensure that having gained our better health and good looks, we keep them for longer too.

5

oils for beauty

There's no doubt that eating the right type of oils improves our health and vitality, but natural plant oils can have a dramatic effect on the skin too. Their benefits are twofold: firstly, eating *vital oils* in our diet or swallowing them in the form of supplements dramatically improves our complexion and helps delay the signs of ageing. Secondly, by applying oils directly to the skin we provide it with many of the nutrients it needs to stay supple and strong. Oils are such effective moisturisers that they are the key ingredients in almost all 'rejuvenating' and 'anti-ageing' skin treatments. Some plant oils, such as wheatgerm, are a wonderfully rich natural source of vitamin E, which neutralises the excess free radicals that cause cell damage. Free radicals are destructive particles that attack the collagen and elastin protein fibres that support the skin, making it look saggy and slack. By using oils that are rich in EFAs and natural source vitamin E (both internally from what we eat and externally from what we apply to our skins) we're able to help promote and prolong a healthy, youthful and radiant glow in two powerful and effective ways.

Natural beauty boosters

The advantages of *vital oils* are not limited to the EFAs that we naturally eat from everyday foods such as fish and olive oil. Many oil supplements, from borage to flax seed, have specific skin conditioning benefits when both taken as supplements and used on the skin in botanical skincare. Plant oils have been highly prized for their skin-softening properties for thousands of years and they were the forerunners of modern skin creams. Today, scientists are rediscovering their secrets and have found that *vital oils* significantly improve the condition of the skin, strengthen nails and give a natural glossy sheen to hair. Some natural oils are good sources of the oil-soluble vitamins such as A, D and E, as well as the EFAs needed by the skin to maintain tone and elasticity. Many natural oils also contain useful amounts of lecithin, the emulsifier discussed on p.68, which also has important water-holding properties. Lecithin can help 'lock' moisture within our epidermal (top layer) skin cells, plumping up parched skin and reducing dryness.

Beauty from within

Taking specific oil supplements on a daily basis can care for our complexions from the inside out and even delay the signs of ageing by slowing down the formation of fine lines and wrinkles. The EFAs found in oils such as evening primrose and borage oil, for example, help strengthen the delicate membranes surrounding skin cells and make them more able to resist attack from destructive enzymes during the ageing process. These EFAs slow the signs of ageing by keeping the skin cells functioning in a healthy way, for longer, and can help cells resist the attacks from the free radicals that lead to cellular disorganisation, skin sagging and wrinkles – not to mention an increased risk of skin cancer. So far, this book has focused on the many health benefits that *vital oils* can bring. But by increasing the amount of *vital oils* in our diets, we can not only improve our health but also improve our looks. No other natural remedy works as well to keep us looking younger, for longer.

The ageing factor

We live in a youth-orientated society, in which teenage models stare out at us from magazine covers and the unlined faces of the young advertise 'anti-wrinkle' remedies aimed at much older women. Before looking at ways of slowing down the ageing process we should first be asking why we feel the need to do so. There's nothing wrong with growing older and the quest for eternal youth is a doomed voyage. A far more realistic approach is the quest for youthful vitality, for a complexion that glows with energy and healthy radiance. This is both more attractive *and* achievable.

The beauty industry is adept at selling a clever blend of hype and hope in a jar, but can anything really make the skin look younger? The answer firstly depends on how you define 'younger looking'. Do you measure the time-lapse in minutes or years? All moisturising creams should temporarily improve the skin's appearance by plumping up the top layer of skin cells, but this action doesn't turn the clock back very far. Many claims are made for reducing wrinkles or making the skin look younger, firmer, etc. However, these results are often measured with extremely sensitive equipment such as electron microscopes that can detect tiny differences barely noticeable to the naked eye.

The more extreme options, such as collagen and botox injections, work for a limited length of time but are temporary, extremely expensive and come with side-effects, including the possibility of facial paralysis – and no one really knows the long-term implications of injecting these substances (and their preservatives) directly into the bloodstream. Fortunately, there's a safer and more natural way to help slow down the rate of skin ageing and encourage a healthy, glowing complexion. That is to look at what is happening beneath the skin's surface and help support the creation of fresh, new skin cells from within.

HOW THE SKIN AGES

To understand the ways in which *vital oils* can help it is worth getting to grips with how the skin works and why it ages. The skin is the largest organ in the body and weighs 2.7–3.6kg (6–8lb). Its function is to hold our insides together and protect internal organs from daily hazards such as bacteria and chemical pollutants. Skin is also the body's thermostat, regulating body heat through perspiration while excreting toxins and waste-matter via the pores. Our skin also prevents us from literally drying out! It does this by producing its own form of oil called sebum in the numerous sebaceous glands that lie just beneath its surface. These glands continually secrete sebum, whose function is to keep the skin moist and supple. So, although our skin may look static it is in fact constantly on the move, continually shedding dead skin cells and replacing them with fresh, young ones. These new cells are produced in the lower level of the skin called the dermis and take around 28 days to travel their way up through the different layers of the outer skin, or epidermis, to reach the surface. The fact that the skin cells are renewed every month means that changes to our diet and skincare regimes can be seen on our faces within four weeks.

Many things influence the way our skin ages. These include hereditary factors that determine the genetic structure of our skin and lifestyle factors such as stress, smoking, alcohol and diet. It has been said that we should choose our parents very carefully … Of all these variables, diet is probably the most important and certainly the easiest to change. Skin needs a rich supply of several vitamins and EFAs to keep it in good condition, all of which can be found in *vital oils*. Plant oils are naturally rich in vitamin E, the most famous skin vitamin. This nutrient is often referred to as the vitality vitamin because of its repairing and regenerating properties within the body. Other vitamins, such as A and D, and EFAs are also important.

Vitamin E for the skin
Vitamin E has the Latin name tocopherol, which comes from *tocos* meaning 'birth' and *phera* meaning 'to give', so its meaning is to give birth or life. Vitamin E occurs naturally in plants, where it primarily helps to protect the oil-rich seed from rancidity, which is why some seed-oil crops are the richest source of this vitamin. The concentrations vary between plants, and are generally high, with the exception of coconut and palm kernel oils, which only contain traces of vitamin E.

Vitamin E is an antioxidant, so it is able to prevent cell damage from destructive free radicals. These particles are a normal byproduct of the body's metabolism, but in excess they can multiply out of control and damage healthy tissue. Free radicals also contribute to the ageing process by destroying the collagen and elastin fibres that support the skin. Without their support our skin slackens and loses its youthful firmness. In addition, free radicals interfere with the formation of fresh, healthy skin cells, making our complexion blotchy and dull. Vitamin E has the ability to neutralise free radicals as soon as they are formed and will help prevent this trail of damage. Its action as a free radical scavenger has led to its being a common skincare ingredient.

However, not all vitamin E is the same. The natural source vitamin E (d-alpha tocopherol) is more powerful than the synthetic variety (dl-alpha tocopherol) and should always be used in preference. The chemical structure differs between the two, with the natural form being more than twice as potent within the body. When buying supplements, look for the description 'natural source' on the pack. Alternatively, check the small print for its description. An easy way to remember which type to buy is that *d*-alpha = delivers vitamin E; *dl*-alpha = delivers *less* vitamin E.

Research shows that vitamin E can help improve moisture levels, improve our natural protection against UV radiation from the sun and delay the progression of skin ageing. Vitamin E is also able to speed wound healing, decrease the depth of fine facial lines, reduce the signs of age or 'liver' spots on the skin and improve overall elasticity. However, the value of vitamin E as a nutrient first became known, not to delay premature ageing, but to help prevent a variety of cancers, cataract formation, arthritis and heart disease. Some of the most exciting studies in this regard, carried out at both the Cardiovascular Research and Medical Statistics Unit in Edinburgh and the Vitamin Unit at Berne University in the 1980s, have shown vitamin E to be valuable in protecting against cardiovascular disorders. Low levels of vitamin E were found to increase the risk of developing angina (chest pain) dramatically. One member of the medical team, Professor Michael Oliver, says that some populations with a high incidence of coronary heart disease may benefit from eating diets rich in natural antioxidants, particularly vitamin E, so there may be a great deal to gain from adding this important supplement to our daily diet. Most supplements of vitamin E contain 100–400IU (international units), equal to around 60–250mg depending on the type of vitamin E used.

Vitamin A for the skin

Another important vitamin found in some animal fats and oils, such as cod liver oil, is vitamin A (also known as retinol). The body needs this nutrient to maintain healthy eyes and vision as well as to repair skin tissues. Vitamin A controls the rate at which skin cells are shed and replaced by new ones. A shortage of vitamin A leads to a sluggish turnover of cells and a sallow, scaly complexion. Vitamin A deficiencies may also lead to the condition hyperkeratosis, where the fresh, young cells die before they reach the skin's surface, resulting in a dry, flaky complexion. This flaky skin tissue then accumulates with sebum and diet to form spots and pimples, and can lead to more serious skin disorders such as acne and dandruff.

Although vitamin A is found in animal produce, notably cod liver oil, it can also be converted by the body from its vegetable forerunner, beta carotene, which version is found in colourful fruits and vegetables, such as carrots – hence its name carotene. Most supplements of pure vitamin A (retinol) contain between 2500mcg and 6000mcg. However, as excess vitamin A is stored in the liver, pregnant women and young children are seldom advised to take retinol supplements. As beta carotene supplements are water-soluble and so not stored within the body they are a safer option. Those who are concerned can switch from taking cod liver oil to an alternative fish oil supplement that does not contain high levels of retinol.

Vitamin D for the skin

Vitamin D is the third oil-soluble nutrient. It is found in animal fats, cod liver oil and in synthetic form in margarine. Vitamin D is also created by the skin through the action of sunlight. In fact, as little as 10 to 15 minutes of midday sunlight on our arms or legs two or three times a week can supply all the vitamin D we need. Vitamin D is needed for healthy skin and skeletal development and works with calcium to build strong bones and teeth. It also affects the quality and tone of skin tissues and promotes healing, which is why it is used in ointments for burns and abrasions. Children who do not get enough vitamin D can develop the bone deformity rickets and low levels of vitamin D in adulthood can also lead to osteomalacia, a bone disease that most commonly appears in women during the time of the menopause. Most vitamin D supplements contain 200–400IU (international units), or 5–10mcg, but a deficiency is rare. Those at risk of a deficiency include the elderly or housebound, who do not have the chance to absorb the sun through their skin. In these cases, a daily dose of cod liver oil (see p.17) can supply several different nutritional benefits.

Essential fatty acids for the skin

The skin needs more than vitamins, though, in order to slow the signs of ageing. The omega-6 EFAs are also required to build the membranes that surround every skin cell and to strengthen the protective lipidic barrier (oil-rich layer) that lies beneath the surface of the skin and guards against moisture loss. A diet deficient in essential fatty acids soon shows up in the face and one of the side-effects of a low-fat or fat-free diet is a dry, devitalised complexion. In the short-term this is not too much of a problem, although parched skin adds years to the face. But starving the skin of EFAs for long periods of time can lead to serious skin problems and premature ageing. In addition, low levels of certain omega-6 polyunsaturated fats (such as GLA) reduces the strength of the skin's supporting collagen fibres, may slow wound healing and can even trigger hair loss. The only way to ensure we receive generous supplies of these important EFAs is to opt for the beneficial *vital oils* that give us these beauty as well as health-giving properties.

Vital oils on the skin

Although natural oils are important ingredients in sophisticated skin creams, their use in beauty treatments is nothing new. Oils have been highly prized for centuries for their therapeutic skincare effects and one of the earliest recorded uses of oil on the skin is in the New Testament. 'Mary took a pound of costly spikenard and anointed the feet of Jesus' (John 12:3). This simple gesture was, in fact, the height of extravagance as spikenard was an extremely expensive, aromatic oil from the remote valleys of the Himalayas. It was extracted from the tiny roots of the fragile spikenard plant and this amount would have cost the average worker an entire year's wages.

Another ancient oil found in the Bible is cassia oil, produced from cinnamon trees. Cassia oil is extracted from cinnamon bark and was mixed with olive oil, which was in plentiful supply around Palestine. The resulting blend was used after bathing to keep the skin soft, smooth and sweetly scented.

In Ancient Egypt, Queen Cleopatra was famed for the amount of time she spent beautifying herself and her narcissistic regime included face masks and massage lotions made from these nourishing seeds. An Egyptian stone carving in at Deir-el-Bahari shows a woman applying oil to her hair, and in the temple of Hatshepsut at Thebes there are paintings of high-ranking Egyptian women having their shoulder massaged with aromatic oils. This treatment was revived in the twentieth century and renamed aromatherapy, and it remains a highly effective way of conditioning and caring for the skin.

Pure, unrefined oils have certainly withstood the test of time and scientists have yet to improve on their ability to protect and repair the skin. Despite many millions of pounds spent on research and development by the cosmetic industry each year, these natural oils remain some of our most valuable and versatile skincare assets.

A–Z of oils for beauty

The following *vital oils* have useful skin caring properties when used on the skin, either on their own or in special facial or body massage blends (see Carrier Oils, p.120).

ALMOND OIL (*Prunus amygdalus*)

Almond oil for health and beauty can be traced back for centuries. The type of oil used for beauty preparations is warm-pressed from sweet almond kernels and is sometimes referred to as 'sweet almond oil'. The earliest use of almond oil in this country was during the Roman occupation, when it was first introduced to Britain. It was obviously a great success as almond oil continued to be an important element of skincare throughout medieval times. In 1372, the Queen of France is recorded as ordering 227kg (500lb) of almonds with the sole purpose of extracting their oil for her face creams. Later, Napoleon's Josephine ran up equally extravagant bills for 'crème amande' which she used as a hand cream and moisturiser. Almond oil was a favourite beautifier throughout Europe and in Britain the 16th-century herbalist John Gerard wrote, 'oil of almonds makes smoothe thye hands and face of delicate persons and cleanseth the skin from spots and pimples.' Almond oil was also the base for the famous traditional hair tonic, Macassar oil, which consisted of almond oil scented with cassia extracts.

Almond oil is a useful source of vitamin E and is traditionally associated with strong, healthy nails. One of the simplest nail treatments is to warm a few drops of almond oil in the palms of your hands before massaging it around the base of the nail and cuticles. The cosmetics industry is still a major purchaser of almond oil – it is added to a great number of modern, emollient formulae, from hair conditioners to hand creams. Unrefined almond oil is available from health food shops and chemists and is a useful ingredient for massage blends. Those with sensitive skins should also see Nut oil allergies, p.69.

APRICOT KERNEL OIL (*Prunus armenaica*)

Apricot kernel oil is similar in structure to peach kernel oil, except that it is higher in polyunsaturates. However, for beauty purposes, it has the same light texture and can be used in exactly the same way. The apricot tree is small and twiggy with an abundance of white flowers tinged with red that appear at the beginning of spring. Its botanical name comes from the Latin word *prunus*, meaning 'plum' and it is a member of the plum family. Apricot trees flourish in temperate climates and were first noted in Armenia and China. While the apricot fruits are rich in beta carotene, the vegetable precursor to vitamin A, the oil comes from the seed kernel and contains only traces of nutrients. However, apricot oil does contain useful levels of essential fatty acids. It also has a wonderfully light texture, making it very easily absorbed into the epidermis or uppermost levels of the skin.

ARGAN OIL (*Argania spinosa*)

Argan oil comes from the seeds from the *Argania spinosa* – an ancient tree that originally grew many thousand years ago across much of Morocco. Following the Ice Age, most of the argan trees died, leaving only a small area in the arid desert region close to the Sahara desert. The argan now only grows in the area of Haha (originally in Argana, a village north-east of Agadir) in southern Morocco, although there are some experimental plantations in Israel. The argan tree is known as the Tree of Life and the oil it produces is known locally as the Gold of Morocco. The local Berber people have many uses for argan oil, from anointing newborn babies to providing fuel for lamps. They also use it as cooking oil, a hair pomade and massage oil for skincare. In fact, argan oil has special properties that make it especially valuable for skincare in their scorching hot, dry climate.

Argan oil is one of the richest natural source of alpha-tocopherol, one of the chemicals that belong to the vitamin E family of tocopherols. This nutrient is especially important for its antioxidant action and is also responsible for the good storage stability of the oil. Unfortunately, argan oil is only produced in limited quantities and, as it comes from a remote region of Morocco, is both difficult to find and expensive. As well as natural vitamin E, argan oil also contains beta carotene and traces of other nutrients. Its unique combination of ingredients includes a rare group of plant sterols considered to be highly effective at helping to heal scar tissue, reduce inflammation and help repair sun-damaged skin. These plant sterols may even have a role in helping to prevent skin cancer. Studies show that argan oil can help improve skin cell function, stimulate cellular renewal and help neutralise the formation of the free radicals that are the primary cause of premature skin ageing.

AVOCADO OIL (*Persea americana*)

Avocado oil is a traditional beauty oil that was used by the tribeswomen of Mexico and Arizona. The oil comes from the flesh of the avocado and was one of the easiest vegetable oils for early civilisations to extract. The avocado tree was first found growing in South America swamplands and still carries the nickname Alligator Pear. It is a distant relative of the magnolia and bay laurel, and grows in California, Mexico, Florida and Mediterranean countries. The Aztecs were the first fans of this fruit and claimed it to be an aphrodisiac. Other cultures used avocado oil for more medicinal purposes and in the Philippines it was sold as a cure for conditions as diverse as toothache and dysentery. In the early 16th century the Franciscan priest Toribio de Montolinia recorded its use in Mexico and wrote, 'Among the fruits found in the mountains is one they call "achucatl", which hangs on the tree and looks like a large pear. The fruit is so wholesome that it is served to the sick. Water prepared from the broad, green leaf is good as a remedy for the legs and even better for the face.' Since then, avocado oil has continued to be acclaimed for its skincare properties and to be an important ingredient for the cosmetic industry.

Although we mostly use avocado in savoury recipes, it is technically a fruit because it contains a stone. Avocados are highly nutritious, being a good source of monounsaturated fats, lecithin, beta carotene, vitamin E and some vitamin C. Despite their high oil content, they do not contain any cholesterol, but they do contain linoleic acid, the parent of GLA. Avocado oil comes from the exceptionally oily flesh of the fruit, which consists of up to 30 per cent pure oil – a figure rivalled only by the olive and palm fruit. Crude avocado oil is produced by mechanical pressing on hydraulic presses, followed by centrifugal extraction. It is not usually extracted using solvents. Although the oil is monounsaturated it is not as stable as olive oil at high temperatures and so not as suitable for cooking. In its crude state, avocado oil contains large amounts of chlorophyll that colour it a dazzling shade of emerald green.

Avocado oil is a time-tested skin soother and softener, but scientists are only beginning to realise its full skincare potential. Research carried out in the USA has revealed that avocado oil not only smooths the surface of the skin but can also penetrate its uppermost layers. Clinical trials have shown avocado oil to be more easily absorbed by the skin than other well-known cosmetic oils such as olive and sweet almond. By carrying its vital vitamins and EFAs below the surface of the skin, avocado oil could play an important part in delaying skin degeneration and help slow the signs of ageing.

A few vegetable oils are also natural sunscreens – and again avocado beats the other beauty oils in its ability to block out the sun's rays. Studies show that the oils most able to block the sun's harmful rays are (in order) avocado, sweet almond, sesame, safflower, coconut and olive. As the sun's rays are our primary cause of premature skin ageing, avocado oil is a useful additional ingredient in facial moisturisers. Avocado oi is highly compatible with all but the most sensitive skin types and, while research into its exact scientific properties goes on, it is clearly one of our most valuable botanical skincare ingredients.

BORAGE OIL (*Borago officinalis*)

One of the most recent natural oils to be used in skincare is borage oil. This oil can help improve the appearance of the skin, not only from within when swallowed, but also when applied directly to the skin's surface. One of the signs that the body is having problems converting linoleic acid into GLA is a dry, flaky complexion. This can be for many reasons. It may be that the body isn't getting sufficient supplies of GLA from the diet, or that the conversion process is being hindered by viral infection, alcohol, smoking or hereditary factors. While a daily internal dose of borage oil (or evening primrose oil) can significantly improve the look and feel of dry skin, the capsules can also be pierced and the contents rubbed into the skin (alternatively you may be able to find a liquid version of borage or evening primrose oil in a dropper bottle). The GLA in these oils will be absorbed by the uppermost layers of skin cells and can help prevent a loss of moisture.

Borage oil provides the richest source of GLA and is probably the best choice to use directly in creams and oil blends on the skin. However, the unique structure of evening primrose oil means that it may be a better choice for treating inflammatory skin conditions (see Eczema, p.44). Because they both are relatively sticky, concentrated oils, it is easiest to mix them with another lighter oil, such as grape-seed or apricot kernel. This blend then forms a protective layer on the epidermis and helps to keep the complexion supple and strong.

CASTOR OIL (*Ricinus communis*)

Castor oil is a natural oil that is better known for its powers as a laxa-tive than for its effect of the skin. However, it is used in protective hair and skin products. Castor oil comes from the castor plant, which is native to West Africa and Mediterranean countries. It is a small, thorny shrub with blue-green leaves and tiny pink flowers that cluster along its spiky stems. An attractive shrub, the caster oil plant also makes a decorative indoor plant. The castor beans lurk beneath the profusion of flowers and contain its many hundreds of glossy brown seeds. These seeds are extremely poisonous if swallowed and so the plant should not be used in houses or gardens where small children might be tempted to eat its berries. However, the oil that is extracted and puri-fied from them is very useful in the world of health and beauty as it is a good natural waterproofing agent. Its lubricating and water-repelling properties are used in a wide range of formulations, from hair shiners to babies' nappy rash creams. Castor oil is also found in some hair lacquers and can be blended with other emollients to make barrier creams. It is used in many ointments for sensitive skins and also has the ability to clear red eyes, which is why it can be found in eye drops.

The castor oil plant features in herbal medicine as a laxative and is now widely grown for its oil, which is also used on a wide scale as a commercial lubricant. Many old wives' tales surround the purgative effects of castor oil and it is reputed to have the ability to induce labour. As a last resort measure for overdue babies, some midwives still suggest knocking back half a glass of castor oil mixed with orange juice (to make it slightly more palatable). However, there is little evidence that this piece of folklore actually works.

COCONUT OIL (*Cocos nucifera*)

South Sea islanders are renowned for their long, dark glossy tresses and smooth, sun kissed skin – despite the fiercely drying effects of the tropical sun. One of their beauty secrets is coconut oil, which is extracted from the dried flesh of the coconut. This dried flesh is called copra and it contains an extraordinary amount of oil, about 65 per cent on average. Coconuts are the fruits of the hardy palm tree that thrives on dry, sandy soils. The tree is a botanical giant, growing over 15 metres (50 feet) high with leaves that measure up to 1.82 metres (6 feet) long. The fragrant white coconut flowers lead to the huge fruit that can weigh over a kilo (2.2lb) each and are enclosed in a hard protective shell. Coconut oil is an important ingredient in the beauty business and is mainly used in soaps and natural cleansers. It has a gentle, low-lathering cleansing action that is less irritating to the skin than chemical detergents. Coconut oil can also be used by itself and the Tagai women of the Philippine Islands comb it through their long black hair to give it a high-gloss shine. It is also an excellent base for body massage oil blends (see Carrier oils, p.120). Coconut palms grow on many tropical coastlines and the principal oil-producing countries are the Philippines, Malaysia, Sri Lanka and Indonesia.

EVENING PRIMROSE OIL (SEE BORAGE OIL)

JOJOBA OIL (*Simmondsia chinensis*)

Jojoba (pronounced ho-ho-ba) oil comes from the jojoba shrub grown in tropical America, notably Southern Arizona, Southern California and Argentina, and is a valuable natural newcomer to skin-care. The jojoba plant is a hardy evergreen that grows 0.6–1.82 metres (2–6 feet) tall with small dark brown beans. It is one of the few plants that thrive in arid, desert regions and can withstand the fierce climatic conditions of strong winds, fierce heat and prolonged drought. The oil is extracted from the beans, and technically speaking, is more of a wax than oil as it is solid at room temperature. Traditionally reputed to be a hair restorer, jojoba oil is one of the most popular natural emollients for skin and hair conditioning in natural cosmetics as it can be used instead of petroleum waxes.

Jojoba is another of our botanical beauty assets and has a long-standing traditional use by the American Indians in Mexico and Arizona where the beans grow wild. Jojoba oil is valuable because it requires little or no refining and has several specific skincare properties. Its chemical composition is close to the skin's own oil, sebum, making it good for all skin types. Because of its natural affinity with the skin, jojoba oil is especially good for sensitive complexions, or oily and acne skin conditions that require delicate treatment. When massaged into the skin, it combines with sebum and gently unclogs pores to help free embedded dirt and grime.

Although jojoba oil is naturally solid, it melts at body temperature, producing a firm texture for skin creams, yet swiftly melting when rubbed on the skin. It also has unusual anti-bacterial properties that help it to resist spoilage and rancidity. Jojoba oil is relatively stable at high temperatures and is less prone to oxidation. This means it has a long-shelf life and will last longer than some of the other plant oils.

Jojoba oil is prized as a cruelty-free ingredient as it is a vegetable alternative to spermaceti, the oil of the great sperm whale. Its use was developed during the 1970s when the whale became listed as an endangered species. Technically, spermaceti is neither an oil nor a fat, but a waxy substance from the head of the sperm whale. This gruesome extract used to be a common ingredient in moisturisers, where it was used for its skin-softening properties. It was added as a cosmetic ingredient to thicken skin creams and give them a glossy shine. Both cheap and highly emollient, spermaceti featured in skincare products from the late 1700s onwards. Fortunately, however, spermaceti and other whale imports are banned in Europe, the USA and most other enlightened nations. Jojoba oil has played an important part in helping to reduce the worldwide demand for whale oil and an extensive planting programme has been carried out in many developing countries. As these crops come to fruition, they are securing the future of some of the world's poorest people – and the great sperm whale.

NEEM OIL (*Azadirachta indica*)

Extracted from the crushed leaves and seeds of the neem tree, neem is sometimes incorrectly classified as an essential oil. The tall, majestic neem tree is a close relative of the hardwood mahogany and is indigenous to Southern India where it grows in tens of millions. An important part of traditional Indian medicine, its name in Sanskrit means 'reliever of sickness'. Neem trees are often found growing outside the door of Indian homes as the leaves and seeds have very useful insect-repelling properties. As an example, swarms of locusts will strip most trees bare, but leave the neem untouched. However, neem does not appear to affect beneficial insects, such as bees and ladybirds, and is not toxic to humans. The quality of neem oil can vary enormously – at the time of writing it may be priced for the trade anywhere from £4 to £100 per kg.

Neem contains more than 35 biologically active principals and has many medicinal properties. It is anti-bacterial, insecticidal, anti-fungal and anti-inflammatory. Neem is also an extremely useful remedy for headlice as its main insecticidal ingredient, azadirachtin, appears to block the cell growth and reproduction of insects and so it will eventually kill them. Neem oil is also used in Indian medicine to help treat skin disorders, including eczema and psoriasis. Studies have shown neem to be both anti-irritant and anti-inflammatory. One study has even showed neem oil to be four times more effective than hydrocortisone.

Neem oil has a distinctively pungent aroma and would not be a first choice for blending unless you are looking for a therapeutic essential oil to help a particular problem. A few drops of neem oil mixed into sweet almond oil makes a useful treatment and preventative remedy for headlice. This blend can also be successfully used to treat fungal infections, including ringworm and athlete's foot. Burning or diffusing the oil will deter insects and provide a distinctively antiseptic aroma. The pungent aroma of neem can be disguised somewhat by blending with spice and citrus oils.

OLIVE OIL (*Olea europea*)

Olive oil is mankind's original skin soother and was the very first oil used in beauty treatments. As described on p.73, its health benefits are far ranging, but it also plays an important part in caring for the skin. The cosmetic benefits of olive oil have been recognised for thousands of years, and it was originally used by the Ancient Greeks and Egyptians for body massage. A useful source of vitamin E, olive oil is wonderfully soothing and can help to take the heat out of sore, inflamed skin. The Ancient Greek 'father of medicine', Hipprocrates, prescribed olive oil for sunburn and it is still a useful after-sun soother. Olive oil has a rich, slightly sticky texture and can be combined with lighter oils, such as grapeseed or apricot kernel for massage blends (see Carrier oils, p.120). Its power as an emollient is recognised by the medical profession and purified olive oil is used in hospitals to treat chapped and scaly skin conditions. My first daughter was born two weeks late and with severely dehydrated skin. The first thing I was given was a tiny bottle of purified olive oil with which to massage her and within days her skin was as smooth and soft as a baby's should be! As well as softening the skin, olive oil also makes a useful hair conditioner. As with most plant oils, it helps increase the tensile strength of the hair shafts making them more elastic and less likely to split or snap. Its rich texture is especially suited to giving body and shine to slightly coarse, thick hair. A few drops combed through the ends of very dry hair will also help to tame frizzy, fly-away ends.

PASSIONFLOWER OIL (*Passiflora incarnata*)

The passionflower is a herbaceous perennial plant native to South America that was later cultivated all over the Mediterranean. It was introduced to Britain from Brazil in the 17th century and grows in gardens on the south coast of England or under glass elsewhere in Britain. The passionflower takes its name from the stunning purple-tinged yellow or pink flowers that are said to resemble Christ's crown of thorns from The Passion (the twelve stages of the cross). The flowers have a group of central filaments or 'corona' that resemble the crown of thorns, while the stigmata are in the shape of the cross with the stamens representing the nails. The flowers give way to large orange berries called passion fruit that are roughly the size and shape of a small apple. Inside the passion fruit's hard outer casing is a soft yellow pulp that contains a mass of shiny, hard black seeds. Passionflower oil is warm-pressed from these seeds and is not usually extracted with solvents. It contains a high percentage of linoleic acid, the parent of GLA.

The leaves and flowering tops of the passionflower have very different qualities from the oil and are used by herbalists as antispasmodic relaxants. American physicians who used the herbal *passiflora* extract in the field of neurology first noticed these seductive properties in the late 19th century. *Passiflora* extract is a narcotic, with a similar chemical composition to morphine. The extract is often combined with other calming herbs such as scullcap, hawthorn and valerian to make powerful sedative brews. *Passiflora* extract is the main ingredient in a German sleeping pill called Vita-Dor, commonly prescribed for treating insomnia. It is also found in many UK herbal medicines, such as Natracalm, and a patent has even been issued for a sedative chewing gum that also contains *passiflora* extract. Other medical uses for the herbal *passiflora* extract are for helping to treat bronchitis, asthma and as a topical treatment for burns, where herbal compresses containing the extract appear to reduce inflammation. The passionflower oil itself does not have any sedating or anti-inflammatory properties and is principally used in beauty treatments for its fine texture and, when in its unrefined state, as a food supplement for its high levels of essential fatty acids.

PEACH KERNEL OIL (*Prunus persica*)

Peach kernel oil originates from China and is another ancient oil reputed to have been brought to Britain by the Romans. The oil comes from the peach kernels of the *Prunus persica* tree, easily recognised in springtime by its mass of bright pink flowers. Peaches need plenty of sunshine to ripen and are ready for picking towards the end of the summer. The fruits are then sliced open prior to canning, while the kernels are cold-pressed to yield the oil.

Peach kernel oil is a pale golden colour and has a light, sweet smell. When used on the skin it sinks easily into the upper levels of the skin, making it a natural favourite for facial massage. Peach kernel oil is high in both mono- and polyunsaturates and can be taken as a supplement to help promote hair texture and shine. It also contains useful levels of vitamin E, making it a useful topical oil to encourage skin suppleness and elasticity. Peach kernel oil is increasingly available in its natural, unrefined state and is an excellent botanical ingredient for facial and body massage blends (see Carrier oils, p.120).

ROSEHIP OIL (*Rosa rubiginosa*)

Also known as *Rosa mosqueta* or muscat rosehip seed oil, the natural oil from these seeds has a high content of useful fatty acids as well as beta-carotene, bioflavonoids, vitamin C and trans-retinoic acid, a form of vitamin A. This last ingredient could be responsible for some of its remarkable therapeutic properties within the skin. Rosehip oil is also high in unsaturated fatty acids, including linoleic and (more unusually) alpha linolenic acid, part of the omega-3 family. These are essential in the defence mechanisms of skin cells as well as other biochemical processes related to tissue regeneration. Rosehip oil is probably the most effective plant oil for restoring healthy skin and clinical studies have proven its ability to help heal scar tissue, reduce 'age' pigmentation spots and improve the appearance of fine surface lines. An excellent addition to facial massage blends or it may be used neat to help problem areas such as scarring.

SESAME OIL (*Sesamum indicum*)

The sesame plant is another native of southern Asia and the Mediterranean, and also has a long association with botanical beauty. The plant itself is a leafy shrub scattered with pinkish white flowers. It requires several months of constant, hot sunshine to ripen the seedpods that contain its seeds. Sesame oil is extracted from these seeds, which can contain up to 60 per cent pure oil. Sesame oil has been used for thousands of years in beauty treatments and was widely used by the Ancient Egyptians, Greeks and Romans. It has a fine, light texture and almost no smell, making it an ideal base for blended massage oils. Sesame oil is a useful natural source of vitamin E and the minerals calcium and potassium. It also contains a small amount of natural sun screening properties, helping to prevent low levels of ultra-violet radiation from damaging the skin. However, sesame oil's natural sun screening properties are not sufficient to protect the skin from damage from strong sunlight. Sesame oil is monounsaturated oil and, like olive oil, is less likely to become rancid in the heat. It also has a longer shelf-life than some of the other polyunsaturated plant oils.

WHEATGERM OIL (*Triticum vulgare*)

Wheatgerm oil is another *vital oil* with a long and noble history. Traces of it have been found in Egyptian tombs dating back to 2000 BC and in prehistoric lake dwellings in Switzerland. Wheat Is one of the world's most important foods and is the largest crop grown in Britain today. Wheatgerm oil is extracted by warm-pressing or solvent expression from the 'germ' of wheat. It is extremely rich and nour-ishing, is one of our richest sources of vitamin E and also contains low levels of some of the B-complex vitamins. Because of its high vitamin E content, wheatgerm oil is a natural antioxidant and is well protected from the elements that usually break down vegetable oils, such as light and heat. Wheatgerm oil is too rich and sticky to use on its own, but it is very useful when added in small amounts to other oils to boost their nutritional value and help protect against rancidity. Wheatgerm oil can help improve the condition of dry, more mature complexions and is a useful addition to facial massage blends. Its drawback is a slightly sour smell that is best disguised with a few drops of aromatic essential oils.

essential oils

*'Fragrant oil brings joy to the heart and
a friend's support is as pleasant as perfume'*
Proverbs 27:9

Fewer natural extracts are shrouded in more myth and magic than essential oils. Don't be put off by the technical jargon and usage warnings that sometimes accompany them, as essential oils are not only a delight to get to know, but also essential everyday beauty and health remedies.

Essential oils are highly aromatic natural extracts that have been described by the more poetic as the 'spirit' or 'soul' of a plant. For the more prosaic, an essential oil is a complex mixture of naturally occurring chemicals that scientifically work in different ways. Essential oils come from the tiny oil glands or sacs found in almost all plants. Each root, leaf or flower oil has its own unique fragrance and characteristics. All essential oils have distinctive and unique healing properties that can help to improve wellbeing. For example, one of the most popular essential oils, lavender, is antiseptic, mildly analgesic (pain relieving), antibiotic, decongestant, relaxant, anti-inflammatory and sedative so it has a wide range of uses, from simple beauty baths and massage to helping with sleep disorders and depression.

There are many hundreds of different types of these aromatic essences, extracted from a plant's flowers, leaves, stalks, seeds, roots or rind. The ceaseless rise in their popularity has meant that just about every health food shop, department store and chemist now stocks a selection.

Historical notes

Although hugely popular today, the use of essential oils in beauty and health treatments is nothing new and they have been used by holistic practitioners for literally thousands of years. One of the first recorded uses of essential oils was by an Egyptian called Imhotep, who used them in massage treatments. He went on to be deified by the Ancient Egyptians as a god of medicine and healing. The Ancient Egyptians were also adept at incorporating plant extracts in their everyday life, using perfumed oils, scented barks, resins and spices in food, medicines and even mummification for the afterlife. The first perfumes were not worn on the skin, but burned as incense. In fact, the word perfume comes from the Latin *per fumum*, meaning 'through smoke'.

The use of essential oils in the bath is also long established and as far back as 2500 years ago, Hippocrates found aromatic baths useful in the treatment of a wide range of disorders, and wrote, 'The way to health is to have an aromatic bath and scented massage every day.' All essential oils are antiseptic to a greater or lesser degree – a fact known in 1800 BC by the Babylonians, who used myrrh, cypress and cedarwood oil to ward off infections. They even perfumed the mortar with which their temples were built – an idea, perhaps, for today's construction industry? Later, the Ancient Romans continued to add drops of sweet-smelling essential oils to their famous Roman baths and huge amounts of frankincense, benzoin and myrrh were burned in their many temples.

The use of essential oils as medicines started to decline as scientific drug research began to replace traditional plant medicine and over time much has been forgotten. However, the use of these aromatic healers continued to crop up from time to time throughout history. During the 13th century, France became an important perfume centre and was the world's leading producer of floral essential oils such as rose and jasmine. Even though diseases such as yellow fever were rife at the time, the perfume workers were rarely affected, and it is thought that the antiseptic qualities of the oils protected them. Studies have since shown that the micro-organisms responsible for yellow fever are easily killed by contact with essential oils. During the great influenza epidemics of the last century, it was also noticed that those who worked in the spice factories (notably cinnamon) were far less likely to succumb to the rigours of infection. This may have been due to their inhalation of these natural antiseptics.

Apart from their medicinal properties, many essential oils were produced solely for their fragrance. The famous French essential oil production for the early perfumers centred mainly around Grasse, a town situated high in the hills in the South of France, where the abundant sunshine and well-drained soil suits the fields of exotic flowers needed to make fine fragrances. Grasse was originally a tannery centre, and the perfumers sold their wares to the leather-workers who made fragranced gloves. In the 18th century bathing was deemed to be unhealthy and so no one took much notice of personal hygiene. As a result, fragranced gloves were popular amongst the gentry to mask the smell of body odour. Nowadays essential oils are produced all over the world, but Grasse still has a reputation of producing some of the finest floral extracts.

The French connection

Although the therapeutic powers of essential oils have been known for thousands of years, it was not until 1937 that they were scientifically analysed. The man credited with cataloguing their medicinal proper-ties was the French cosmetic scientist, René-Maurice Gattefossé, who coined the term *aromathérapie*. Gattefossé first realised the healing potential of these oils after he badly burnt his hand during a laboratory experiment. To relieve the pain he is reputed to have plunged it into the nearest vat of liquid, which happened to be lavender oil. Gattefossé was amazed at how quickly the oil soothed his inflamed skin and helped it to heal. He went on to detail large numbers of essential oils and discovered that many were more effective healers than their synthetic counterparts. Another Frenchman convinced of the powers of essential oils was the Parisian army surgeon, Jean Valnet. During the Second World War, Dr Valnet used essential oils as antiseptics to treat war wounds. He also noticed that the troops who slept rough in the dense pine forests suffered from fewer respiratory infections. Recognising that the aroma from the pine trees was the active ingredient, Dr Valnet used essential oils as the focus of his work. When the war ended, Valnet wrote *Aromathérapie*, published in 1964, which is now published in English (*The Practice of Aromatherapy*) and has become an aromatherapist's almanac.

The French are far more accepting of the powers and therapeutic properties of essential oils and there are several medical schools that include the study of essential oils as part of their curriculum. A form of herbal medicine called phytotherapy is widely practised across Europe today and this also features the use of essential oils. A look in the many currently published scientific, medical and cosmetic journals reveals an increasing interest in the therapeutic properties of essential oils, from simple beauty treatments involving scented oils for relaxing massage to the topical application of powerful skin healers.

Extracting essential oils

Although they are termed 'essential' these highly concentrated extracts should not be confused with the edible omega-6 vegetable and omega-3 fish oils that contain essential fatty acids and vitamins. Here we are talking about the odorous, volatile extracts of a single plant that consist of carbon, hydrogen and oxygen atoms. These are chemically quite distinct from edible fats and oils and should not be eaten! Essential oils can come from any part of a plant and the term 'volatility' often applied to them simply means that they will evaporate if left open to the air. Interestingly, different essential oils can be extracted from different parts of the same species, such as the orange tree, whose flowers yield neroli oil; leaves and twigs produce petitgrain oil; and fruit rind produces orange oil.

ENFLEURAGE

The oldest method of extracting essential oil is enfleurage and this is still one of the best methods of obtaining the oil from fragile flower heads such as jasmine. Within hours of picking, the flowers are placed on sheets of glass that have been covered with purified animal fat or beeswax. As the oil from the flowers soaks into the fat, so more layers of petals are added until the fat is completely saturated with essential oil. This traditional method of production is often carried out in sheds beside the flower fields for maximum freshness. I witnessed this process one summer in Grasse, from dawn-picking of the flowers through to the soaking of the petals at dusk, when the intensely sweet, almost sickly aroma of the blooms hangs heavy in the warm night air. This method of extraction particularly suits jasmine blossoms, which continue to release their aroma for 24 hours after picking. The fragrant mulch produced at this stage is called a 'pomade' and was originally used in its raw state as a gentleman's hair dressing. To release the oil, the pomade is dissolved in alcohol and the fat sinks to the bottom of the container. The mixture is then heated so that the alcohol evaporates, leaving the pure essential oil behind. The enfleurage extraction process is still carried out by hand and is much more time-consuming than other more mechanised methods. Even collecting the raw materials is highly labour-intensive. It's estimated that it takes a staggering 8 million jasmine flowers to produce a single kilo of pure essential oil this way. Not surprisingly, jasmine is one of the world's most expensive fragrant essences.

DISTILLATION

As romantic as enfleurage sounds, it must be said that these days most essential oils are extracted by the more high-tech methods of distillation. The Arabian herbalist Avicenna probably invented this method in the 11th century. During alchemy experiments using rose petals, Avicenna discovered that if the flowers were placed in a flask and heated, the vapour could be collected in another flask. Avicenna identified this fragranced vapour as rosewater and the substance floating on its surface as pure rose essential oil. The modern process of distillation involves combining the aromatic part of the plant with boiling water or steam. The vapour then travels along a series of glass tubes that form a condenser. The essential oil droplets are siphoned off through a narrow-necked container and the remaining water collected in a container below. The essential oil may then be filtered before bottling. Distillation is by far the most common extraction method and works well for most essential oils, including the exquisite rose otto.

Hydrolats

Hydrolats are the naturally perfumed waters that are produced during the distillation process (they are not water to which a few drops of essential oil have been added). A hydrolat is created as the essential oil vapour mixes with the steam during distillation. The vapour separates as the steam cools in the condensing tank, separating the essential oil molecules from the steam. This then cools to become water and the essential oil floats to the surface, creating two separate layers: the upper layer is the essential oil, which is filtered or siphoned off, and the remaining delightfully scented water is called the hydrolat, or hydrosol. The hydrolats produced from flowers are called 'floral waters' and contain similar volatile components to the pure essential oil but not quite as strong. Their chemical composition is also different as they are soluble in water, unlike essential oils, which only mix with other oils. Useful antiseptic and anti-inflammatory substances are found in many hydrolats and they are becoming increasingly popular as natural skincare ingredients.

SOLVENT EXTRACTION

Technically speaking, the process of solvent extraction yields 'absolutes' and not pure essential oils. It is a method used by the perfume industry primarily to release the fragrance from flowers and can be a less expensive method of extraction. Solvent extraction is a highly mechanised procedure and some aromatherapists believe that the end product is devitalised and lacking in therapeutic properties. Nevertheless, the absolutes that are produced are a natural product and often have a superior fragrance, hence their popularity with the perfume industry. Solvent extraction begins by mixing flower petals together with a solvent using rotating paddles that encourage the petals to release their oils. After several hours the petals are strained off, leaving a mixture of solvent and perfumed 'absolute' behind. To retrieve the absolute, the mixture is heated so that the solvent evaporates away. The process is labour-intensive, as the blooms must be picked by hand – and it takes approximately 6000kg (15,2300lb) of petals to produce a single kilo (2.2lb) of rose absolute.

Choosing the method of extraction is often more to do with what the resulting essential oil is going to be used for. Steam distillation is the preferred choice for maximising therapeutic properties, while solvent extraction usually produces a superior aroma. Rose, orange blossom, frankincense and mimosa are the most common absolutes produced by solvent extraction.

EXPRESSION

Citrus oils such as lemon and mandarin are more easily (and cheaply) available and are extracted by a process called expression. In the good old days, the rinds of the fruits were squeezed by hand to extract the oil from the multitude of tiny glands visible in the peel. As with the rest of life, the process is now highly mechanised and the fruit is first crushed before being placed in a centrifugal extractor. This rotates at high speed to spin out the droplets of essential oils. Simple but effective. However, the problem with expressed citrus oils is that they can retain chemical compounds that cause photosensitivity on the skin when exposed to ultraviolet light. For this reason, most essential oils produced for aromatherapy or cosmetic uses are steam-distilled.

How essential oils work

Essential oils are highly versatile healers and can be used in many different ways. They can be diluted for face and body massage, added to a bath, burnt to give off an aroma, inhaled from hot water, used in a compress or in some cases even applied neat in small quantities on burns and scars.

Essential oils provide the basis of aromatherapy, which literally means 'treatment with aromas'. The woman credited with bringing aromatherapy within reach of the public was Madame Marguerite Maury. This French biochemist with an interest in beauty therapy worked with Dr Jean Valnet and is responsible for bringing aromatherapy as we know it to Britain. It is she who recognised the value of applying oils to the skin using specific massage techniques and developed the holistic principles behind aromatherapy today. Based at her London clinic she not only trained beauty therapists but also nurses, physiotherapists, medical herbalists and doctors seeking alternatives to conventional drug treatments. Aromatherapists who trained under Madame Maury include Micheline Arcier, Shirley Price and Daniele Ryman. These women are now amongst the doyennes of the aromatherapy world and have their own clinics, training facilities and ranges of essential oils.

Many of the newer aromatherapy organisations are also well respected. Aromatherapy Associates is held in high regard and has one of the most attractive and holistic clinics I've come across. Under the direction of Geraldine Howard it also runs some of the best additional courses for trained aromatherapists around the world. Further details of accredited courses or how to find a well-qualified aromatherapist in your area can be found in the Useful Resources section on p.207.

There are two parts to aromatherapy: the first is the smell of the oil and second is the action it has on the body. Our sense of smell is the most powerful of all our senses and has a dramatic effect on the way we feel. It is controlled by the olfactory organ situated above the nose, just below the base of our brain. This organ is covered with a thin sheet of membrane housing approximately 800 million nerve endings, which are there solely to detect smells and are so tiny that they can barely be seen under a powerful electron microscope. Whenever we catch a whiff of something, our olfactory nerves send scent messages to the limbic system in the brain. This is responsible for controlling our moods and emotions and explains why the aromas from essential oils can have such a profound effect on the way we feel. The limbic system is capable of remembering many millions of different smells and nothing evokes a memory faster than a specific smell. There may also be additional chemical components within essential oils that act on the brain – and it is well known that certain drugs act extremely quickly when sniffed up the nose.

Research carried out at the Institute of Pharmaceutical Chemistry, University of Vienna, in 2001, revealed that when the chemical limonene (found in all citrus oils including grapefruit, orange and neroli) is inhaled, systolic blood pressure rises and people report increased feelings of alertness and restlessness. Another chemical constituent in essential oils is carvone (found in dill and galbanum essential oils) and this was also shown to raise both heart rate and diastolic blood pressure. Researchers suggest that prolonged inhalation of chemicals such as these can effect both our autonomic nervous system as well as our mental and emotional state of mind. As well as stimulating the brain, some components in essential oils have been found to have a calming effect. The activity of mice exposed to linalool (found in lavender and camphor) decreased by 40 per cent and failed to increase even after stimulation with caffeine. So it may be that it takes more than a strong cup of coffee to restore our mental agility after a relaxing aromatherapy treatment.

DO ESSENTIAL OILS PENETRATE THE SKIN?

Because they are so powerful, essential oils are usually diluted before they're used on the skin and a few drops in a spoonful of plant oil, such as grapeseed, will be enough to cover the entire body. Most of the constituents of essential oils have a very small molecular structure which some say enables them to 'slip' through the network of surface skin cells and end up in the bloodstream. This may well not be true.

Aromatherapists also like to say that the hands-on pressure of massage further increases this dermal absorption. However, scientists hotly dispute this statement. Medics (including those who specialise in skin permeability) say that no amount of 'rubbing in' can push a substance through such an impenetrable barrier as our skin.

Experiments using essential oils have shown that within half an hour of being applied to the skin, traces of essential oil appear in the urine. How much of the essential oil enters our system from inhaling the aromatic vapours and how much from direct penetration through the skin is far from clear, however. Most experiments showing aromatherapy massage results in terms of traces of essential oil within the body did not exclude the volatile vapours that are inevitably inhaled into the lungs during the treatment. Sitting in an essential oil bath may result in traces of the oils being detected in the bloodstream, but these are likely to have come via inhalation. Frances Fewell, an aromatherapy consultant and educator, and pathway leader for the BSc (Hons) in Complementary Medicine at Anglia University, conducts some of the best studies on the subject. In one, she assessed 100 volunteers, dividing the group into two. The first group received an aromatherapy foot massage using a 2.5 per cent dilution of sweet orange essential oil. The second group also received the same foot massage, but wore airtight breathing apparatus throughout the treatment – provided by the local Fire Brigade! Blood samples were taken at various intervals under sealed-skin conditions to ensure that none of the volatile oils could contaminate the testing. Her initial assumptions that essential oils do not penetrate the skin appear to be valid, although final results are still outstanding at time of writing.

Other, simpler studies have suggested that essential oils can penetrate the skin of mice, but since the epidermis of a mouse is not as complex as ours, these results are not statistically significant. The example of a cut clove of garlic rubbed on the soles of the feet and then being smelt on the breath is also flawed. Garlic has a very different chemical composition to any essential oil and, if you try it for yourself, you'll find that it's hard to avoid inhaling garlic's very volatile vapour while trying out this experiment.

A leading expert in skin penetration, Professor Jonathon Hadgraft, who directs the Skin and Membrane Transfer Research Centre at Medway Sciences, NRI, University of Greenwich, is one of many scientists who believe that the amount of an essential oil that can get through the skin and into the body is likely to be very small and almost impossible to measure. Professor Hadgraft points out that the skin is a highly complex organ that contains layers of both water loving (hydrophilic) and oil loving (lipophilic) materials. The constituents of essential oils tend to be very lipophilic and almost insoluble in water. It is possible for the oils to combine with the lipophilic regions of the skin but very difficult for them to cross the hydrophilic layers. Compounds that cross the skin well, and even then do so very slowly, are materials that have good solubility in both oil and water. The reason why it has taken so long to develop medicinal patches for drug delivery such as HRT or nicotine patches is precisely because the skin is so impenetrable. In general, Professor Hadgraft's research shows as little as 1 or 2 per cent of skincare products overall gets through the skin to the bloodstream, despite many unsubstantiated claims to the contrary.

Our skin has evolved over time to prevent foreign materials from entering the body and for minimising water loss from the body. Without this barrier function we would have skin like frogs and have to live most of the time in water. However, it *is* possible to reduce the barrier function of the skin and some pharmaceutical patches contain special agents to promote percutaneous absorption – ethyl alcohol, for example, can be used to promote the absorption of some compounds. Yet another reason why essential oils are unlikely to end up in the body via the skin is that some of their constituents can be broken down by enzymes within the skin and therefore do not reach the bloodstream intact; for example, esterase enzymes in the skin break down the benzyl acetate in jasmine oil, so a pure jasmine essential oil cannot end up in the body simply by massaging it into the skin.

All the evidence suggests that essential oils do not, in fact, penetrate the skin. However, this does not reduce the value of aromatherapy, it simply changes the mechanism by which it works. Studies show that whether inhaled via the essential oil vapour or absorbed through the skin, essential oils are excreted from the body in breath, perspiration and urine. So it is perfectly possible that they could have a therapeutic effect within the body, especially upon moods and emotions controlled by the brain. And even if some essential oils do penetrate the skin to a small extent, the good news is that there is no evidence of overdose from using a few drops in the bath or for body massage, even for small children or during pregnancy. Whatever your view, essential oils are wonderful to use in aromatherapy and for many beauty and health treatments. The powerful effects they can have on the brain, together with many anti-bacterial and anti-inflammatory qualities, make them potential healers in many ways. In addition, the sheer pleasure of their aroma together with their undoubted powers to uplift, relax and inspire cannot be denied.

Massage oils

When using essential oils on the skin they must first be diluted. Essential oils do not dissolve in water but they do dissolve in oil, so they need mixing with a 'carrier' oil to disperse them on the skin. There are two steps to making a massage oil: choosing which kind of carrier oil will make the best base for your particular blend and then selecting your essential oil. In terms of carrier oils, grapeseed oil has a fine, light texture and is popular with aromatherapists for body massage oils. Sunflower and safflower oils are also light textured, while corn oil is a little too sticky and has a slightly unpleasant smell. For facial massage, I prefer using blends of rosehip, argan, jojoba, avocado, hazelnut, peach and apricot kernel oils as carrier oils. They are more expensive, but only need to be used in small quantities as a little goes a very long way. I also add a few drops of wheatgerm oil to some massage blends. Wheatgerm is rich in vitamin E, an excellent natural antioxidant, and will help protect the oils from rancidity. Alternatively, the content of a natural source vitamin E capsule works well and will smell less stongly.

All massage oils should be both organically grown and/or unrefined where possible to retain their important skin-nourishing nutrients. It's worth looking out for officially organically certified oils, as these have stricter standards of refining and are likely to be less processed. The reason I don't use 'baby oil' is that this can be a mineral oil – an environmentally unfriendly byproduct of the petrol industry. Mineral oil lacks useful skin-nourishing nutrients such as vitamin E and beta carotene and is designed to sit on the surface of the skin, leaving traces of greasiness. Most baby oils also contain synthetic perfumes and I prefer to use naturally scented essential oils that have their own therapeutic benefits.

Carrier oils

Many of the plant oils that make useful carrier oils have already been discussed in detail in the A–Z of oils for beauty, pp.95–107, so the following is more of a quick guide to the specific properties of carrier oils suitable for making massage blends. These carrier oils are safe for all skin types, but it is advisable to patch test first before making up the blend. A small number of people with highly sensitive complexions can develop an allergic reaction even to natural oils, so it makes sense to test each one you use on a small area of skin 24 hours before applying it to the whole body. If you have highly sensitive skin it would be wise to test each new bottle on opening, as natural oils can vary from batch to batch. When preparing oils for the face, it's even more important to only use pure, high-quality – preferably organic – oils and to patch test before use.

ALMOND OIL (*Prunus amygdalus*)
Clear and virtually odourless, sweet almond oil is a slightly sticky oil that is especially suited to body massage blends. Good for most skin types, including dry, easily irritated facial complexions. One of the more stable carrier oils, it can also be stored in cold conditions without clouding. Use on its own or blend with other nourishing oils such as argan or avocado.

APRICOT KERNEL OIL (*Prunus armeniaca*)
A clear, slightly yellow carrier oil with a non-greasy feel; the light texture of this oil is especially suitable for facial massage blends. Good

for more mature, dry, sensitive or inflamed skins. It is an expensive oil to use on its own, so blend with almond, grapeseed or safflower oils.

ARGAN OIL (*Argania spinosa*)

A wonderful oil for facial and body massage as it is light yet naturally rich in vitamin E. Used in the Moroccan *hammams*, or Turkish baths, for massage it has a good, robust texture for body oil blends. The plain, un-toasted version makes a wonderful (if expensive) addition to facial massage blends.

AVOCADO OIL (*Persea americana*)

Excellent for facial massage blends as it temporarily plumps up fine lines and wrinkles. This oil suits most sensitive skins and may help relieve the dryness and itching of eczema and psoriasis. May also be listed as *Persea gratissima* on ingredients labels. An expensive oil to use on its own, so blend with other carrier oils such as almond if required.

BORAGE OIL (*Borago officinalis*)

Also known as starflower, borage oil is a very useful addition to blends for helping skin disorders such as eczema and psoriasis. Because of its GLA content, regular use also helps to encourage younger-looking skin when used in facial blends as it helps to reduce trans-epidermal water loss, restoring skin smoothness and flexibility. Expensive to use neat, the easiest way to use borage oil is to pierce a capsule and add the contents to your facial or body massage blend.

COCOA BUTTER (*Theobroma cacao*)

This soft butter-like emollient is semi-solid at room temperature and is more of a vegetable fat than an oil. However, it can be blended with essential oils and is very popular in some tropical countries for massage. Cocoa butter melts on contact with the skin and provides a lovely base ingredient for face or body massage formulations. It lasts well in hot, humid conditions and is even reputed to have some mild natural sun-screening properties. Makes a useful natural skin salve for areas of extreme dehydration, such as the hands and feet. It has the sweet, pungent smell of chocolate that you either love or loathe, although this can be masked by other more fragrant essential oils. Pure cocoa butter has a reputation for helping to fade stretch marks and heal scar tissue, but rosehip oil is probably a better choice for this.

COCONUT OIL (*Cocos nucifera*)

This oil comes from the coconut palm and is usually only available in its fractionated form, which means that the liquid oil has been sep-arated from the more waxy part of the coconut fruit. The fraction-ated oil retains useful fatty acids and is a good base oil for body massage, giving an easy 'slip' across the skin. Coconut oil suits most skins although it benefits from additional oils being included in the massage blend to boost its nutritional and therapeutic value.

EVENING PRIMROSE OIL (*Oenothera biennis*)

Well-known for its skin-caring properties, cold-pressed evening primrose oil is excellent for adding to face and body massage blends, especially to combat dry, devitalised skin or to help with mild forms of eczema. Expensive (and a bit sticky) to use on its own, so add a few drops or the contents of one or two capsules to your massage blend.

GRAPESEED OIL (*Vitis vinifera*)

A favourite with aromatherapists for its light texture and lack of smell, grapeseed oil is pale yellow in colour and virtually odour-free. Non-greasy and excellent for body massage blends, it suits all skin types. As it is virtually impossible to buy a completely unrefined version, it helps to add other less refined oils richer in vitamins and EFAs to boost its nutrient content.

HAZELNUT OIL (*Corylus avellana*)

This oil is reputedly slightly astringent, so is often recommended for making blends for oily or combination skins. Hazelnut oil has reduced in price in recent years and tends to be a good value, high-quality option for many massage blends.

JOJOBA OIL (*Simmondsia chinensis*)

This wonderfully light carrier oil is a good base for some facial oil blends as its fine texture is suited to oily and combination skin types. It penetrates the upper levels of the skin more easily than most oils and is also useful, if expensive, for body massage.

MACADAMIA OIL (*Macadamia ternifolia*)

Usually cold-pressed and then refined, macadamia is another nut oil with an excellent texture for massage that soaks easily into the epidermis. One of the most penetrating, it is sometimes called the 'vanishing oil'.

MEADOWFOAM OIL (*Limnanthes alba*)

A relative newcomer to aromatherapy blends, the texture of this oil is similar to jojoba oil and when added to blends it is a superb natural skin moisturiser, leaving behind a healthy gleam.

OLIVE OIL (*Olea europaea*)

This oil is easily available in its cold-pressed, unrefined state. However, it does have a slightly sticky texture and so suits dryer skins. Excellent for adding to body massage blends and for soothing sore, chapped skin. Purified olive oil is available in small bottles from the chemist and is recommended as the first massage oil for tiny babies, as it is unlikely to cause sensitivity.

PASSIONFLOWER OIL (*Passiflora incarnata*)

A useful, natural source of vitamin E and trace minerals, passionflower oil helps maintain skin elasticity and is an excellent addition to face and body massage blends. Although expensive, it is an excellent addition to fine facial blends.

PEACH KERNEL OIL (*Prunus persica*)

Choose carefully from a reputable supplier as this oil is sometimes mixed with other kernel oils, such as almond or cherry before bottling. A useful source of essential fatty acids, vitamin E and traces of some minerals, peach kernel oil is a very good addition to face and body massage blends. It has a useful element of beta carotene if not over-refined and can be used as a substitute for apricot kernel oil. Helps prevent skin dehydration and is especially suitable for more sensitive complexions.

ROSEHIP OIL (*Rosa rubiginosa*)

Also known as *Rosa mosqueta*, rosehip oil is probably the most effective plant oil for tissue regeneration and clinical studies have proven its ability to help heal scar tissue, reduce 'age' pigmentation spots and improve the appearance of fine surface lines. It makes an excellent addition to facial massage blends, or, alternatively, can be used neat to help problem areas such as scarring.

SAFFLOWER OIL (*Carthamus tinctorius*)

Another favourite with aromatherapists for body massage because of its light texture and penetrative power. It is also virtually odourless and so is useful for blending with subtly scented essential oils. Safflower is also one of the least expensive and most readily available oils and can be found on almost all supermarket shelves.

SESAME OIL (*Sesamum indicum*)

Unrefined sesame oil contains good levels of vitamin E and lecithin, and is excellent for adding to facial massage blends.

SHEA BUTTER (*Butyrospermum parkii*)

Not a carrier oil as such, but a useful natural emollient for blending with other plant oils and essential oils, this greyish, waxy substance comes from the pressed fruits of a typical African Savannah tree. Shea butter is a soft natural fat that melts at body temperature, making it an interesting and unusual ingredient for body massage. It has similar skin benefits to cocoa butter, without the same chocolatey smell. Shea butter contains small amounts of naturally anti-inflammatory allantoin and clinical studies report good skin soothing properties for chapped, sun burnt and irritated skins. Pure shea butter is also reputed to provide low levels of natural sun screening.

WHEATGERM OIL (*Triticum vulgare*)

Natural wheatgerm is bright orange in colour with a strong, pungent odour. Darkly aromatic, this oil is too sticky to use on its own but makes a wonderful addition to dry skin massage blends. Those who find wheatgerm oil too pungent to use can substitute it with pure vitamin E oil, as this has no odour.

Blending oils

Having chosen your carrier oils, the next step is to select which essential oils to add. You'll find a full A–Z of essential oils on p.131. Essential oils are highly concentrated so should be used sparingly. As a rough guide you need approximately 1 drop of essential oil for every 5ml of carrier oil. Once blended, the massage mixture should be stored in a cool, dark place. A friendly chemist will sell you the small amber glass bottles they use for medicines and these make the best containers. Alternatively, see Useful Resources on p.209 for details of the best professional suppliers. Some bottles also come with their own glass or plastic pipettes which are useful for accurately measuring small quantities of oil. This book is not about recipes so much as about giving you the knowledge and freedom to have fun creating your own oil blends. However, for the first-timers among you, here are a few of my own personal tried-and-tested home favourites. For ease of reckoning, 5ml = 1 teaspoon.

Balancing facial massage blend

An excellent all-rounder to balance most skin types.

> 25ml (1fl oz) peach or apricot kernel oil
> 25ml (1fl oz) jojoba oil
> 5 drops wheatgerm or 1 natural source vitamin E capsule
>   contents
> 1 borage oil capsule contents
> 5 drops lavender, 3 drops rose-scented geranium, 2 drops neroli
>   essential oils

Plumping-up facial oil

Wonderful for temporarily filling out fine lines and restoring moisture to parched skins, this soothing blend may also be helpful for Acne rosacea. Use last thing at night and as often as required. If you have difficulty finding all the oils, this blend is similar to Superbalm Concentrate, from Liz Earle Naturally Active Skincare, details of which can be found in Useful Resources, p.203.

    25ml (1fl oz) avocado oil
    10ml (2 tsp) argan oil
    10ml (2 tsp) rosehip oil
    2 borage oil capsule contents
    1 natural source vitamin E capsule contents
    3 drops sandalwood, 2 drops neroli, 2 drops rose essential oils

For help with eczema

Anything applied to damaged skin must be patch tested first and used cautiously for the first few times in case of an adverse reaction. I have found this blend helpful for my children too. Apply sparingly after bathing with a chemical detergent-free cleanser, such as Liz Earle Orange Flower Botanical Body Wash.

    50ml (2fl oz) purified sweet almond or olive oil
    5 borage or 10 evening primrose oil capsule contents
    5 natural source vitamin E capsule contents
    5 drops organic chamomile essential oil

For help with problem skins

Hormonal skin conditions such as adolescent acne and persistent spots respond well to a night-time application of purifying, antiseptic oils. Use sparingly, avoiding eyes and lips.

    50ml (2fl oz) jojoba or hazelnut oil
    4 drops lemon tea tree, 3 drops cypress, 3 drops lavender
        essential oils

Skin-saving body oil

Perfect for moisturising after bathing or to use as a home massage blend.

    50ml (2fl oz) grapeseed or coconut oil
    50ml (2fl oz) passionflower oil
    3 borage oil capsule contents
    5 drops lavender, 3 drops lime, 2 drops ginger essential oils

De-tox hip and thigh formula

Similar to the Liz Earle Energising Body Gel treatment (which also contains organic rose water and botanical extracts) which was formulated with the help of essential oil specialists, Aromatherapy Associates. Use twice a day on areas of sponginess (hips, thighs, ankles) to help improve blood flow and circulation.

    100ml (4fl oz) grapeseed or safflower oil
    4 drops each of grapefruit, rosemary, pine, juniper, petitgrain
       and peppermint essential oils

Bath oils

Adding essential oils to the bath is one of the easiest methods of enjoying their many benefits – and their wonderful aromas turn bath-time into a whole new sensory experience! Essential oils are quickly broken down by heat, so make sure the bath water is warm, not hot. Add the oils after the bath has run, then dim the lights, step in, relax and enjoy. As a general rule, 5-10 drops of essential oil should be sufficient. Children love fragrant baths and this is an easy way of using well-diluted essential oils on their delicate skins. Babies, too, have a keen sense of smell and appreciate aromatherapy treatments – just one drop of a floral essential oil (such as chamomile or lavender) is all that's needed for an aromatic baby bath.

Burning and diffused oils

Essential oils were the world's first air fresheners and they are certainly more ecologically sound than chemical-laden plug-ins or sprays. Oil burners are now widely available and most health shops sell ones that are heated with night light candles. The top half of these burners should be filled with water to which a few drops of essential oils are then added. The drawback to this type of oil burner is that it can get extremely hot and the water quickly evaporates, leaving behind a blackened residue of burnt oil. Also, it is not advisable to leave a naked flame unattended at any time. Electric oil burners – consisting of a smooth ceramic surface that heats up at the flick of a switch – make good high-tech alternatives. The essential oils are dropped on to the top and kept at a constant temperature – just hot enough to release the vapour without risk of burning. Safe, simple and clean, electric oil burners are ideal for offices and children's bedrooms.

Other modern methods of burning oils include fragrance rings. These are ceramic or cardboard discs that balance over the top of a light bulb. The essential oils are dropped on to the ring and the warmth from the bulb releases their aromatic odour. The problem with using burning rings is that many essential oils (notably frankincense and pine) have low flash-points and so are highly flammable. Cardboard and porcelain rings can get very hot if placed for many hours on an illuminated bulb, so should not be left unattended in case of fire. Also, don't be tempted to drop essential oils directly onto the light bulb as this can shatter the bulb.

Burning essential oils is a useful way to fragrance the atmosphere, but keep in mind that heating an essential oil can dramatically alter its chemical structure. To retain the therapeutic properties of an essential oil, you will need to use a cold dispersal method (diffusing). This means that the pure vapours of essential oil are pumped out into the atmosphere without first being burnt. A good way of releasing pure essential oil vapour into the atmosphere is to use glass diffusers. These consist of a small electric air pump connected to an intricate series of glass tubes. When filled with neat essential oils, the pump blows air through the oil and the effect is like a mini-waterfall dispersing tiny droplets of fragrant oil into the atmosphere. A glass diffuser should be used for about 20 minutes every few hours and some models can disperse oil into quite large areas such as hospital wards. Glass diffusers are used therapeutically in hospices and some cancer patients have found the aroma of citrus oils beneficial as they remove the depressing institutional smell. Plastic plug-in electric oil diffusers are also available and these work by placing the essential oils onto an absorbent pad and allowing a small motorised fan to whirr the vapours into the room. Although easier to obtain, I have not found these to be as efficient as the glass diffusers.

Inhaling oils

The rejuvenating power that essential oils possess is easily demon-strated by inhaling them. Just a few drops of eucalyptus oil sprinkled on to a tissue will instantly clear a stuffy head, while a drop or two of lavender oil on the fingertips rubbed across the temples revives and invigorates. The easiest way to inhale oils is by sprinkling a few drops on to a tissue that can then be tucked in a breast pocket or shirt-sleeve. A few drops can also be dabbed on to pillows to induce a good night's sleep (I always travel with a bottle of lavender oil to help me sleep when away from home). Don't use essential oils directly on clothing, however, as they can stain wool, silks and other delicate fabrics.

Additional methods of inhalation include adding a few drops of essential oil to a basin of hot water, covering your head with a towel and breathing the vapour in deeply. This is particularly effective for clearing a chesty cold as the hot steam helps ease congestion. My own favourite inhalation blend for this is made from equal quantities of eucalyptus, pine, rosemary and clove or ravensara essential oils. I make up a bottle in the autumn for the family's inevitable winter colds and it really does work wonders.

Compress oils

The French are fond of using compresses to treat numerous skin complaints and some of the best results are seen on conditions that involve bruises and swelling. To make a compress you will need an absorbent material such as a muslin cloth, flannel, cotton wool or lint. Dip this into a small bowl of warm water containing 10–20 drops of an essential oil. Next, wring the material out so that it is damp but not dripping and apply it to the affected area. To prevent the essential oil from evaporating, wrap clingfilm around the entire area and cover with a warm towel. Ideally the compress should be left in place for at least an hour. Lavender essential oil is one of the most useful for making compresses.

Neat essential oils

Although essential oils are mostly used well-diluted there are a few occasions that merit using them directly on the skin. Neat lavender oil, for example, is wonderfully soothing on burns, minor scrapes and grazes and I keep a bottle handy in the kitchen for this very purpose. Lavender oil also reduces subsequent burn scarring and can dramatically speed up the healing process. All essential oils are anti-septic and have many applications in first aid. Just one drop on the skin will take the initial sting out of insect bites and nettle rash. A blend of lavender and lemon tea tree can also be used neat in tiny quantities on stubborn spots, boils and pimples. Use a clean cotton bud to apply, avoiding lips and eyes.

Pure melissa (lemon balm) also has therapeutic properties and many swear by dabbing a tiny dot on to the first sign of a cold sore. Although melissa is sometimes classified as a skin irritant, most aromatherapists agree that it is both well-tolerated and useful in small quantities in dilutions of up to 2 per cent. Neat essential oils should not be used on babies unless under the guidance of a well qualified aromatherapist – and always wash your hands after use to avoid inadvertently rubbing essential oil into your eyes.

Internal use

Essential oils are too potent to be taken internally without an extremely thorough knowledge of the subject. Some aromatherapists, however, do prescribe the internal use of diluted essential oils for a very few, specific disorders. These are usually taken in the form of one or two drops in a glassful of water. Essential oils should only be used in extremely small quantities and, given the potentially toxic nature of some oils, it is important to be guided by a qualified practitioner.

Essential oils are used as flavourings by the food and drink industry, but in relatively small amounts. For example, almost all toothpaste and mouthwash is flavoured with peppermint oil, as are many peppermint sweets. Aniseed, fennel, dill, eucalyptus and pine are all used as flavourings for confectionery and pharmaceutical products, from cough lozenges to children's linctus. Earl Grey tea was originally simply China tea flavoured with a few drops of bergamot essential oil. This oil give the tea its pungent taste and was named after the Englishman Earl Grey, who remarked on its unusual flavour while visiting a Chinese mandarin in the 19th century. Sadly, most Earl Grey teas are now made with a synthetic chemical equivalent to the natural essential oil. Some aromatherapists advocate using a drop of other highly aromatic oils such as jasmine and peppermint to flavour tea, but you do need to be sure of what you are drinking! In this case, it is even more important to buy essential oils from a trusted and reputable professional supplier, as the market is unfortunately rife with adulterated and mis-labelled essential oils.

A–Z of essential oils

BASIL (*Ocimum basilicim*)
Source: Leaves and flowering tops from the herb. Native to Europe.

Background: From the Greek *basileus*, meaning 'king'. Basil is one of our oldest herbs and has been cultivated in Europe since the 12th century. Traditionally revered in India, where it is regarded as a sacred plant and dedicated to the Hindu gods Krishna and Vishnu, the true sweet basil oil is steam distilled from the flowering top of the herb, whereas the Exotic or so-called Reunion type of basil oil is produced in the Comoro islands, the Seychelles and Madagascar and has a more camphoraceous aroma. Sweet basil oil is the more expensive variety.

Actions: Antiseptic, stimulating, insecticidal.

Properties: A natural tranquilliser with a mentally stimulating effect. One of the best aromatic nerve tonics that can help the body cope under stressful conditions. A powerful oil that can help fight fatigue but an excess can also act as a depressant. The main identified chemical constituents of the essential oil are estragole and linalool, with eugenol, limonene and geraniol.

Uses: The aroma is good at awakening the senses. Burning a few drops while working encourages mental concentration and discourages flies and mosquitoes. Use only as directed by an aromatherapist. Has a toning effect on the skin when used in massage blends and can be used to help combat cellulite. Blends well with other herb, citrus and spice oils.

BAY LEAF (*Pimenta racemosa*)

Source: Leaves from the tree. Native to the Mediterranean.

Background: Bay trees grow wild in the West Indies where their leaves are widely used in cooking. The leaves have a pungent taste and aroma and are especially useful to season fish and meat. Bay leaves are covered in tiny oil glands that release a delicious scent when pressed or shaken by the wind. This aromatic fragrance was especially popular with the Romans who gave bay leaf garlands to army and literary heroes. Bay leaf oil is also traditionally associated with healthy hair and hair growth.

Actions: Antiseptic, uplifting.

Properties: Yellow or dark brown in colour, bay leaf oil is a useful all-round tonic. It has a fresh, spicy and slightly medicinal aroma that was the original base for Bay Rum. Useful for respiratory disorders and used by aromatherapists to help treat depression. Also mixed in to massage blends to treat aches, sprains and rheumatism. The main identified chemical constituent of the essential oil is eugenol, with some linonene and linalool.

Uses: A few drops will make a fortifying bath. Add to scalp oils to discourage hair loss and help improve dandruff. Blends well with other herb, citrus and spice oils.

BENZOIN (*Styrax benzoin*)

Source: Made from the resin obtained by deep incisions into the benzoin tree cultivated in Java, Sumatra and Thailand.

Background: Brought back to Europe from the Orient by the early 17th-century traders. Natural gum is greyish with red streaks and it is the red streaks that contain the most aromatic compounds. Benzoin was used as an antiseptic treatment for respiratory conditions and is one of the classic ingredients of incense. The main identified chemical constituent of the essential oil is benzoic acid.

Actions: Antiseptic, diuretic, expectorant, sedative.

Properties: Best known as the main constituent of tincture of benzoin or Friar's Balsam inhalant. A potent skin sensitiser in its pure resin form, benzoin is not a true essential oil. Perfumes and topical skin treatments containing benzoin should use a far less irritating version that has been modified to remove the skin allergens. The main identified chemical constituents of the essential oil are benzyl cinnamate and benzyl benzoate.

Uses: Not generally used in home care. Modified versions are used by the fragrance industry and blend well with spice, wood and citrus oils. Often used as a natural fixative to prolong a perfume's staying-power.

BERGAMOT (*Citrus aurantium bergamia*)

Source: Rind from the fruit. Native to Italy.

Background: This delicately scented oil is named after the town of Bergamo in northern Italy, where it was originally cultivated. The Ivory Coast now produces most of the world's supply today. The fruit resembles a small orange and has featured in Italian herbal medicine for centuries. The oil is cold pressed from the oil-bearing glands on the fruit's surface and has a deliciously fresh aroma. Bergamot oil is traditionally used to flavour Earl Grey tea (although most manufacturers now use a reconstituted synthetic flavouring) and is a traditional ingredient in eau-de-cologne. Top quality bergamot oil is olive-green in colour that fades with age. The leaves of the *Citrus bergamia* tree can also be used to make bergamot-petitgrain oil, which can be used by the unscrupulous for 'cutting' or diluting pure bergamot essential oil.

Actions: Antiseptic, anti-viral, uplifting, refreshing.

Properties: Useful for treating infected skin conditions such as boils, spots and acne. Aromatherapists may use bergamot oil to treat infections of the urinary tract as it has traditionally been used to help cystitis and urethritis. Pure expressed bergamot essential oil contains bergaptene, a chemical that causes photo-sensitivity if the skin is exposed to ultraviolet light. For this reason it should definitely be avoided during sun exposure and used with caution when outside even on relatively cloudy days. A wiser option is to choose the bergaptene-free oil, known as FCF (furanocoumarnin-free) bergamot. The main identified chemical constituents of the essential oil are linalyl acetate, limonene, linalool and (in some cases) bergapten.

Uses: Add to massage blends for helping to lift depression. Bergamot has an attractive aroma that can improve mood and help focus the mind. Good for burning or diffusing and adding to a relaxing end-of-day bath. Suits combination and oily skin types. Has a longer shelf-life than other citrus oils and can be kept in a cool, dark place for two to three years without serious deterioration. Unlike other citrus oils, Bergamot is a useful natural 'fixative' as it helps prolong the aroma of other oils and it blends well with wood, resin, floral and citrus oils.

BLACK PEPPER (*Piper nigrum*)

Source: Black peppercorns are sun-dried berries cultivated in India, Madagascar and Java.

Background: Black pepper, along with cinnamon and cloves, is one of our oldest spices and has been grown in India and China for thousands of years. Highly prized, black peppercorns were originally used as trade money along the Spice Route in the 15th century. Black pepper berries were first brought to Britain by the Roman Empire and have remained part of our culture ever since.

Actions: Analgesic, antiseptic, digestive, stimulant, tonic.

Properties: Used in homeopathic medicine to help improve concentration and depression as well and wind or colic. Known as a rubifacient, which causes temporary reddening and warming of the skin. Rubifacients are often used as counter-irritants for the relief of muscular pain. The main identified chemical constituents of the essential oil are phellandrene and pinene.

Uses: Works well in massage blends to help muscular aches and sprains. Has a similar scent to clove and blends well with woods and spices, such as sandalwood and ginger.

CAJUPUT (*Melaleuca cajuputi*)

Source: Leaves and twigs from the tree. Native to Indonesia.

Background: Also called the Swamp Tea Tree, this Indonesian tree has small fragrant white flowers that cluster around a long spike. The oil is extremely aromatic and smells rather like tea tree oil (it comes from a similar tree). The chemical composition of cajuput is almost identical to that of eucalyptus, except that it has a milder and sweeter aroma. Cajuput is also very close to niaouli essential oil, which is extracted from the leaves of the *Melaleuca viridiflora* tree. It was traditionally mixed with olive and almond oils to help soothe sunburn.

Actions: Antiseptic, uplifting, restorative.

Properties: Improves mood, increases resistance to infections, especially coughs, colds and flu. Used by aromatherapists to help gynaecological problems including painful periods and cystitis. The main identified chemical constituents of the essential oil are caryophyllene cineole, pinene, geraniol, limonene, linalool and sesquterpenes, including cadinene.

Uses: Add in tiny quantities to stimulating massage blends or to make a therapeutic warming bath. Excellent as a highly aromatic and purifying room fragrance. Add to massage blends for its subtle, soft herby aroma and uplifting effect. Blends well with floral, citrus and spice oils.

CARDAMOM (*Elettaria cardamomum*)

Source: Seeds from the husks of the plant. Native to India.

Background: One of the oldest essential oils known, cardamom oil was used in Eastern herbal medicine for over 3000 years, and by the Ancient Greeks and Egyptians as incense and perfume. Hippocrates wrote that cardamom was useful for massage and the physician Dioscorides prescribed crushed cardamom seeds for abdominal pains and fluid retention. Cardamom oil is used both medicinally and for cooking. It has traditionally been grown in India and Sri Lanka, although India remains by far the largest consumer. Most cardamom essential oil used to be produced in Europe and the USA, but more recent production in India has increased its supply. Good-quality cardamom oil is also produced in Guatemala and this is darker in colour than either the European or American oils. Pure cardamon oil is expensive and some are 'cut' or diluted with cineol to reduce their cost, so always buy from a reputable supplier. Cardamom belongs to the same botanical family as ginger and is used in similar ways for its warming actions.

Actions: Antiseptic, refreshing, invigorating.

Properties: A good digestive aid used by aromatherapists to help stomach disorders, nausea, heartburn, colic and painful bouts of wind. Chewing a cardamom pod often helps to relieve these conditions and improve bad breath. Has a stimulating effect on the body and is used in India as an aphrodisiac. The main identified chemical constituents of the essential oil are limonene, linalool, geraniol, citral and cineole.

Uses: A richly aromatic oil with a pleasantly warm, sweet, spicy aroma that should be used sparingly or else it will overpower other oils in the blend. Useful added to a warm bath to refresh and stimulate the system. As with all spice oils, use with care as it can upset sensitive skins. Blends well with other spice and citrus oils. Cardamom is also used by perfumers to add a richness to floral blends, including geranium and rose.

CEDARWOOD (*Cedrus atlantica*)

Source: Wood shavings from the tree. Native to North Africa and America (depending on the tree).

Background: Because of its wonderfully distinctive aroma, cedarwood was burnt in Ancient Egyptian and Greek temples as incense. The temple of Solomon in Jerusalem, commissioned by David, was built entirely of cedarwood and must have smelt amazing. The amount of wood used for this enormous building was so great that the forests of Lebanon have never fully recovered. Most cedarwood oil used today comes from steam-distilled sawdust and wood shavings from the Atlas mountains in North Africa. Confusingly, cedarwood oil can either come from a pine tree called *Cedrus atlantica* or from cedar trees that are botanically related to the cypress called *Juniperis virginiana* and *Juniperus procera* and others, so look for Atlantic or Atlas cedarwood.

Actions: Antiseptic, diuretic, sedative, insecticidal.

Properties: Used to help respiratory disorders including bronchitis and catarrh. Can help relieve aching muscles and tone the skin. Cedarwood oil is used in many fine fragrances and aftershaves for its excellent aroma. Burning cedar wood chips on the fire is also a subtle way of scenting a room. Many household insects, including mosquitoes, woodworm and moth, are deterred by the scent of cedarwood. The main identified chemical constituent of the essential oil is cedrol.

Uses: Therapeutically similar to sandalwood, only more intense. Has a subtle firming effect on the skin and can be used in oils to help combat cellulite. Suits oily and combination skins and may be added to jojoba oil to help improve spotty skin conditions. Cedarwood is frequently used in perfumery as a natural fixative and it blends well with other woods (such as pine), heavy florals, citrus and spice oils.

CHAMOMILE (*Athemis nobilis, Chamaemelum nobile, Matricaria recutita*)

Source: Dried flowers from the herb. Native to Europe.

Background: Chamomile is named after the Greek for 'ground apple' after the apple-like scent it releases when trodden on. The lawns at Buckingham Palace are laid with chamomile and it is traditionally associated with the nobility. In Elizabethan times, dried chamomile flowers were sewn into small muslin bags and used to fragrance their once-yearly bath water.

Actions: Antibiotic, antiseptic, anti-inflammatory, anti-microbial, anti-fungal, anti-irritant, calming, sedative.

Properties: Several species are grown wild in Europe but only one, *Athemis nobilis*, also known as Roman chamomile, is commonly used for its essential oil. *Matricaria recutita*, found in more eastern parts of Europe and commonly used in chamomile tea, is known as German chamomile or 'true chamomile'. All chamomiles contain a potent anti-inflammatory substance called chamazulene and high levels will give the oil a most beautiful blue colour. Chamazulene is not present in the fresh flowers, but is formed when the essential oil is distilled. The steam generated in the steam distillation process frees the oils and binds with some substances while splitting others, so creating new compounds such as chamazulene, a blue-tinted hydrocarbon, which does not exist in the chamomile plant. Solvent extraction generates more chamazulene, creating an absolute that is a deep ink blue in colour.

Roman chamomile contains about 1 per cent essential oil, whereas German chamomile contains only about 0.25 per cent essential oil. German chamomile is roughly twice the cost of Roman chamomile. Azulene (or, more correctly, chamazulene) is present in both varieties, but tends to be more predominant in German chamomile. Both chamomiles contain limonene and linalool. Roman chamomile also contains small quantities of geraniol. Unfortunately, pure chamomile oil may sometimes be adulterated with *Matricaria suaveolens*, a common weed, or Moroccan chamomile, which comes from a different plant called *Ormenis multicaulis*. Always buy from a reputable source.

Both Roman and German varieties of chamomile provide a gentle, versatile oil that belongs in the first aid, as well as the beauty, box. In fact, chamomile is recognised as a medicinal drug in the pharmacopoeia of 26 countries around the world. It can be used to help nervous conditions, headaches, insomnia, menstrual disorders and skin complaints. Especially recommended for children.

Chamomile tea is useful for regulating digestive disorders and for adding to a baby's bath to soothe sore skin.

Uses: Wonderful in a bath to encourage a good night's sleep. Add to facial massage oils to soothe dry, oily or irritated skin conditions. Look for a naturally blue oil with plenty of anti-inflammatory chamazulene as this is one of the few botanicals that can genuinely help soothe disorders such as eczema. Blends well with other floral, citrus and herb oils.

CITRONELLA (*Cymbopogon nardus*)

Source: The whole plant. Native to Sri Lanka and Africa.

Background: The variety grown in Sri Lanka is steam-distilled from the leaves of the Lanabatu variety of citronella grass. In central Africa, the Java type of citronella (sometimes confused with lemon grass) especially thrives on the dry, stony soil. It is also widely cultivated in Indonesia, China and Brazil. Citronella has an unusually sharp, citrus smell and Alexander the Great is reported to have been invigorated by its scent while riding his elephant through Egypt in 332 BC. Nowadays, citronella is widely used in perfumery, soap-making and for natural insect repellents, as well as for scenting household cleaning products.

Actions: Antiseptic, stimulating, insecticidal.

Properties: Citronella is used in tropical countries as a powerful natural deodoriser. Not commonly used in aromatherapy as it has an overpowering scent and is quite sharp, but it is reputed to boost the immune system and can stimulate a sluggish circulation. Citronella oil from Sri Lanka has a sharply lemon-camphor aroma, whereas the Java variety contains higher levels of geraniol and citronellol which give it a sweeter scent. Both types of citronella oil also contain linolene, citral and linalool.

Uses: A few drops in a massage blend will ward off mosquitoes. If you have been bitten, a small amount can be used neat on stings. May also be used neat to heal minor skin abrasions. An invigorating and refreshing oil for burning. Blends well with other pungent essential oils such as ginger and basil.

CLARY SAGE (*Salvia sclarea*)

Source: Flowering tops and leaves from the herb. Native to Spain.

Background: Also known by the French name *essence sauge sclarée*, clary sage essential oil is steam-distilled from the flowing tops and leaves of the plant. One of the many varieties of sage, clary sage is regarded as less toxic than the common herb, including Dalmatian sage. Clary sage is an attractive plant with large purple flowers and pineapple-scented leaves that carry the essential oil. Traditionally associated with feminine sexuality and gynaecology, clary sage also has euphoric properties and can induce a light-headed feeling. Its soft, pungently herby aroma is not unlike that of chamomile oil.

Actions: Antiseptic, balancing, sedative.

Properties: Contains a hormone-like compound similar to oestrogen that may help to regulate hormonal imbalance. Used by aromatherapists to help pre-menstrual syndrome and symptoms of the menopause. Also used in abdominal and back compresses during labour to help regulate contractions, although the evidence for this is anecdotal. Inhaling the oil or using a few drops in the bath is reputed to help lift post-natal depression. The main identified chemical constituents of the essential oil are linaly lacetate, linalool, with some geraniol and limonene.

Uses: Add to facial massage oils to help problem skins. Excellent for massage blends applied prior to menstruation. Can be burned or diffused as a room essence to improve mood and mental clarity. Over-use can induce a state of euphoric headiness. Blends well with floral, spice, wood and citrus oils, especially coriander, cardamom, lavender, geranium and sandalwood.

CLOVE BUD (*Eugenia caryophyllus*)

Source: Buds from the clove tree. Native to Indonesia.

Background: Clove bud oil is now principally cultivated in Madagascar, Mauritius and Zanzibar (also known as the Spice Island) from the unopened dry flower buds of this tall evergreen tree. Originally distilled as a powerful natural antiseptic and ingredient for incense, clove oil is now also popular amongst perfumers. It may be added to spicy fragrance blends, including many men's aftershaves. Clove oil is also a useful natural insecticide and pomanders made by studding small oranges with cloves can be hung amongst clothes to help deter moths. Cloves are highly aromatic and also have many culinary uses. An aromatic oil may also be extracted from both the leaf and stem of the plant by water distillation.

Actions: Antiseptic, anti-bacterial, anti-fungal.

Properties: Clove bud oil is less irritating on the skin than clove leaf oil, but it is still high in eugenol and aromatic aldehydes that can cause severe skin sensitivity unless used very well diluted. A patch test is especially recommended before use and it is probably best left in the hands of a well-qualified aromatherapist to blend using the correct quantity. Despite this note of caution, studies show clove bud oil to be highly anti-inflammatory and very useful in soothing the skin. Research has also shown clove *leaf* oil to be highly effective against a wide range of bacteria and yeasts, notably *Candida albicans*, but this variety should not be confused with clove bud. Correct labelling is important when purchasing any kind of clove oil, so make sure the label specifies whether it is bud, leaf or stem – and be sure you can trust your supplier to tell the difference!

Uses: Pre-blended, clove bud oil makes a warming and comforting bath blend. Tiny dabs on the end of a clean cotton bud may also help numb the pain of toothache and help to clear minor oral infections. Very small quantities (i.e one drop in 100ml carrier oil) may be included in blends for fragrant bath oils or massage. Blends well with other spices, herb and citrus oils.

CORIANDER (*Coriandrum sativum*)

Source: Seeds of the fruit. Native to Eastern Europe.

Background: Coriander seeds are a well-known Easter flavouring and have been used in herbal medicine for thousands of years. Coriander seeds were found buried beside Ancient Egyptians in their tombs. The name coriander comes from the Greek word *koris*, meaning 'bug'. This is reputedly due to the fact that coriander leaves give off a pungent odour when crushed which reminded the Greeks of squashed bed bugs! Coriander has properties as a *digestif* and was included in the original monks' recipes for Chartreuse and Benedictine liqueurs. An expensive essential oil to produce as the seed contains only 0.7 per cent essential oil, so it takes one metric ton of crushed coriander to yield just 7kg of pure essential oil.

Actions: Antiseptic, calming, analgesic.

Properties: Coriander is a member of the same *Umbelliferae* family as fennel and dill, and has similar properties. It is used by aromatherapists to help with digestive disorders and may help stimulate the appetite. The essential oil has local analgesic properties and can help ease muscular and rheumatic pain. The main identified chemical constituents of the essential oil are linalool, with some limonene and geraniol.

Uses: Coriander is a powerful spice oil and should be used sparingly. It is useful when combined with other oils to make a relaxing bath as it has gently sedative properties. Its warm, sweet aroma blends well with wood, spice, resin and citrus oils – notably neroli, sandalwood and ginger.

CYPRESS (*Cupressus sempervirens*)

Source: Leaves (needles) and twigs from the tree. Native to the Mediterranean.

Background: This large evergreen tree is common in southern Europe where it was planted along the coastline to act as a natural windbreak. The essential oil has a similar smell and properties to pine oil. The first recorded use of cypress oil was about 2000 years ago, when Dioscorides claimed it to be a cure for stomach disorders. Most of the essential oil production centres around southern France and Spain, where it tends to be distilled annually after tree pruning and following the violent Mistral winds, when many twigs and branches are blown off the trees. Pure cypress oil is therefore often limited in quantity and only available at certain times of the year. Despite its scarcity it is not an expensive essential oil.

Actions: Antiseptic, tonic, diuretic.

Properties: A pale yellow oil with a sweet-balsamic aroma similar

FRANKINCENSE (*Boswellia carteri*)

Source: A gummy resin from the bark of the tree. Native to Somalia.

Background: All parts of this tree are highly aromatic but it is the resin that is used to make the essential oil. Most frankincense is solvent-extracted and technically this produces an absolute and not an essential oil. The tree belongs for the *Burseraceae* family, which is divided into many different species, about 12 of which belong to *Boswellia*, the Latin name for the varieties that yield frankincense. Four species are recognised as producing olibanum, which can be inter-changed for frankincense. The name comes from the medieval French word meaning 'real incense'. Frankincense was one of the gifts brought by the Magi to the infant Christ and has been a symbol of divinity for thousands of years. There are two types of frankincense tree in Somalia: the Beyo, which grows out of the ground and the extraordinary Maydi, which grows out of rock. Saudi Arabia is an increasingly important source of frankincense.

Actions: Antiseptic, purifying, expectorant.

Properties: The unusual pungent smell of frankincense helps focus the mind and this oil has meditative qualities. Used to treat stress and nervous tension. The main identified chemical constituents of the essential oil are pinene, phellandrene and verbenone.

Uses: A good oil to burn when overworked or trying to cope under pressure. A few drops rubbed into the scalp help clear the mind and encourage mental stimulation. Suits oilier complexions but is also reputedly useful in facial oils to help deter fine lines and wrinkles. An excellent expectorant when added to steam inhalations or a hot bath. Blends well with spice, floral and citrus oils.

GALBANUM (*Ferula galbaniflua*)

Source: A natural gum-resin. Native to Iran.

Background: Used by ancient civilisations as an incense due to its intense aroma when warmed, galbanum is collected from cuts in the stem of several different species of *Ferula* – large umbelliferous plants from the same botanical family as fennel and dill. Two types of galbanum are produced: soft galbanum for aromatherapy and perfumery, and hard galbanum for the pharmaceutical industry. Soft galbanum yields more essential oil than the hard variety and it has a powerful, green-woody aroma that lingers in the air long after the top has been put back on the bottle! Perfumers liken its aroma to hyacinth leaves and it will invariably be found in hyacinth-based scents. Some aromatherapists store galbanum separately as its aroma can easily contaminate other essential oils.

Actions: Antiseptic, anti-microbial, digestive, warming, calming.

Properties: A very heady oil with a warm, woody aroma that acts as a natural fixative to prolong the fragrances of spice and herb oil blends. Used medicinally as a flavouring for cough medicines and digestive remedies. The main identified chemical constituents of the essential oil are limonene, pinene and cadinene.

Uses: Traditionally associated with dryer skin conditions, galbanum is a useful antiseptic to add to healing massage blends. Also useful added to chest rubs to help improve coughs and other bronchial complaints. May be used by aromatherapists to help treat nervous exhaustion and digestive disorders caused by tension. Also reputed to be an effective pain reliever when used in hot compresses on the skin. Blends well with spice, citrus and floral oils (especially lavender) as it provides a deeply aromatic 'base' for a balanced fragrance blend.

GERANIUM (*Pelargonium graveolens, Pelargonium odoratissimum*)

Source: The whole plant. Native to South Africa.

Background: There are over 700 different types of geranium flower but only a handful are used to make essential oils. The essential oil is steam distilled from the leaves and stems of the *Pelargonium graveolens* and other species of *Pelargonium*, the most sweetly scented being the *graveolens* variety. This has a wonderful, rose-like aroma which comes from an ingredient called geraniol contained in the plant's leaves. These varieties are often referred to as rose-scented geranium and are very important to the perfume industry. Some good quality bourbon-type oil is produced on the small island of Reunion, close to Madagascar and Mauritius in the Indian Ocean, but most of the world's volume comes from China and Egypt. Other producers include the former Soviet Union, which produces about 30 tonnes a year for its own domestic soap production and so rarely exports it.

Actions: Antiseptic, anti-irritant, toning, uplifting, soothing.

Properties: A versatile oil used to help soothe skin irritations and minor skin abrasions. Suits all skin types and is particularly useful for dryer, more mature complexions. Used by aromatherapists to help improve a wide range of ailments including hormonal and menstrual problems. The main identified chemical constituents of the essential oil are citronellol, geraniol, linalool, citral and limonene in varying proportions, depending on the species.

Uses: Can be added to massage oil for its skin-soothing properties and wonderful floral aroma. Suits all skin types including dry, oily and sensitive. Blends well with most essential oils, including citrus, woods, resins, spices and other florals.

GINGER (*Zingiber officinale*)

Source: Roots (rhizomes) from the plant. Native to India.

Background: An important element in traditional Chinese medicine, ginger arrived in Europe via the Spice Route during the Middle Ages. Ginger is used to fight colds and infections, and the Chinese use it to treat any condition relating to an imbalance of moisture such as catarrh or diarrhoea. The essential oil is yellow-orange in colour and has a fresh, herby scent and not the pungent aroma traditionally associated with the root. Ginger has a reputation as an aphrodisiac, and the women of Senegal still weave ginger roots into their clothing to attract the opposite sex. Ginger absolute is frequently used by the perfume industry and may be added to spicy after-shave blends. Popular with the food and drink industry for flavouring many well-known brands, from ginger ale to ginger biscuits.

Actions: Antiseptic, digestive, warming, fortifying.

Properties: Used in massage blends to help improve muscular stiffness and rheumatism. Also used by aromatherapists to help counteract nervous tension and anxiety. Ginger tea, made by infusing a small piece of ginger root in a cup of hot water, is an effective treatment for nausea, especially travel and morning sickness. The main identified chemical constituents of the essential oil are limonene, citral and linalool.

Uses: A powerful spice oil, so use sparingly. Deliciously warming and reviving when combined with citrus oils for a stimulating bath blend. A few drops in hot water make a useful foot bath to help combat colds and flu. Not suitable for very sensitive skins. Blends well with resin, spice, citrus and wood oils, especially sandalwood, vetiver and patchouli.

GRAPEFRUIT (*Citrus grandis*)

Source: Peel of the fruit. Native to the West Indies.

Background: The oil is expressed from the peel of the fruits that are believed to have evolved from the West Indian 'shaddock' fruit. Although not a hybrid, grapefruit is a modern botanical addition as it has only been grown for a hundred years or so, and not in any quantity until the middle of the last century. Cultivated in Asia and the West Indies, grapefruit is now grown mostly in Israel and Argentina. Southern California produces a grapefruit essential oil high in nootketone, an ingredient mainly used as a flavouring for the soft drinks industry. It is also favoured by perfumers for its clean, refreshing aroma and grapefruit essential oil is sometimes used in place of bergamot. Grapefruit seed oil is a powerful natural antiseptic and can be used as a household cleaning agent, a natural preservative and even as a food supplement to help purify the intestines. It is sometimes sold under the trade name Citricidal or grapefruit seed extract and can be found in health shops.

Actions: Antiseptic, anti-bacterial, stimulant, diuretic, tonic.

Properties: A zesty, uplifting essential oil that may be used by aromatherapists to help improve the appearance of cellulite and water retention. Traditionally also used to stimulate the digestive and circulatory systems and its tangy aroma is even reputed to help lessen the appetite. Studies by American researchers have also shown grapefruit essential oil to be anti-irritant on the skin. The main identified chemical constituents of the essential oil are limonene with citral, linalool and (in some cases) bergaptene.

Uses: An ideal addition to stimulating massage blends. Traditionally used to help improve skin tone around the hip and thigh area. Also good as a pre-exercise muscle warm-up rub. Grapefruit essential oil triggers less photo-sensitivity than some other citrus oils, but the expressed essential oil is best avoided immediately prior to sunbathing or sunbeds. The distilled oil should not present a photo-sensitivity problem. Grapefruit essential oil oxidises relatively rapidly once opened, so should be kept cool and dark, and used within 12 months of opening. Suits oily and combination skin types. Blends well with other citrus oils, spices, woods and resins.

HO WOOD (SEE ROSEWOOD)

HYSSOP (*Hyssopus officinalis*)
Source: Leaves from the herb. Native to the Mediterranean.

Background: An ancient flowering herb that receives its first literary mention in the Bible. The leaves produce a highly fragrant oil that is hard to describe – a uniquely fruity, herby aroma. Hyssop is an important ingredient for perfume and several liqueurs, including Chartreuse. It is also used as a food flavouring for pickles, meat sauces and seasonings. Although hyssop is native to Europe it is also widely cultivated in Brazil and the Middle East. Some of the best-quality steam-distilled hyssop comes from Hungary and France.

Actions: Antibiotic, antiseptic, uplifting, tonic.

Properties: Used to help respiratory infections including coughs, colds and flu. Used traditionally by herbalists to help heal bruised skin and regulate high or low blood pressure disorders. Its pick-me-up properties make hyssop especially useful for either body massage or diffusing during convalescence. The main identified chemical constituents of the essential oil are limonene, pinene and pinocamphone.

Uses: An especially powerful essential oil so use sparingly. May be used in compresses for bruised or aching limbs or in small quantities for body massage. Hyssop gives off a warm, vibrant aroma when burned as a room fragrance. Blends well with lavender and citrus oils, rosemary, clary sage and sage.

JASMINE (*Jasminum officinale*)

Source: Flowers. Native to India.

Background: Jasmine is not available as a distilled oil, only as an extremely costly enfleurage oil or absolute, making it one of the most expensive botanical ingredients in the world. Both the enfleurage oil and the absolute are extracted from the palest pink or white jasmine flowers picked by hand annually. It is one of the most important, if not *the* most important, natural perfume raw material and is at the heart of many fine fragrances. Some of the highest-quality jasmine oil comes from Grasse in the South of France, where it has been grown for hundreds of years. However, its production is under threat by property developers building holiday homes on many of the oldest jasmine fields. As there is no satisfactory synthetic equivalent to jasmine, some perfume houses have bought their own jasmine fields to ensure sufficient supplies for their fragrances.

High-quality jasmine is also produced in India where it is cultivated in the subtropical region of the northwest Himalayas. In Indian medicine jasmine is considered good for cooling and softening the skin, as well as to help reduce inflammation. In China, the oil is a reputed anti-depressant and is used in Chinese herbal medicine as a general tonic. The leaves of the jasmine plant contain salicylic acid, an alkaloid helpful in speeding up the removal of dead skin cells. Studies show jasmine oil can also stimulate fibroblast activity within the skin, helping to increase epidermal cell turnover, leading to claims that it may have skin regenerating properties. Unfortunately, as jasmine is a rare and expensive essence it is frequently adulterated with less expensive floral oils, such as ylang ylang, or made synthetically.

Actions: Antiseptic, energising, uplifting, restorative.

Properties: Its intense floral aroma can invigorate and help lift depression. Used by aromatherapists to help improve menstrual disorders, stress and general anxiety. In addition to its exquisitely heady fragrance, jasmine is extremely good for soothing dry, sensitive skins. The main identified chemical constituents of the essential oil are jasmone, linalool, geraniol and nerol.

Uses: An expensive ingredient but one that only needs to be used in tiny quantities. A few drops make a luxurious bath oil. An excellent addition to massage oils for the face and body. Reputed to repair skin tissues and can be used in small quantities to help prevent stretch marks. However, nursing mothers should note that there is some evidence that the smell of jasmine inhibits lactation (this also applies to jasmine in perfume). Suits all skin types. Blends well with other floral oils such as geranium and rose.

JUNIPER BERRY (*Juniperus communis*)

Source: Dried berries. Native to Europe and Asia.

Background: The oil comes from the ripe, dried juniper berries that grow in many regions around the world. The best berries are collected in northern Italy, Austria, Eastern Europe and France. Native to northern Europe, juniper is an increasingly important crop in northern Asia and North Africa. Juniper berries have a pungent, aromatic smell and most juniper berries end up being used to give gin its distinctive, slightly bitter flavour. A wonderful aromatic condiment for many meat dishes, notably pot-roasted lamb. Also a popular component of many after-shaves and traditional eau-de-colognes. A lighter, slightly sweeter scented variety comes from the berries and twigs of *Juniperus smreka*, which comes from Macedonia.

Actions: Antiseptic, anti-fungal, stimulating and diuretic.

Properties: One of the key therapeutic essential oils used by aromatherapists to help improve digestive, urinary and hormonal problems. Its action is similar to that of cypress and, botanically, they are quite closely related. Reputed to stimulate the blood circulation and act as a skin and blood purifier. Studies show juniper essential oil can also stimulate fibroblast activity within the skin, helping to increase epidermal cell turnover. The main identified chemical constituents of the essential oil are pinene, myrcene, terpinen, sabinene and linalool.

Uses: Add a few drops to a detoxifying bath to help relieve tired, aching limbs. Suits oily and combination complexions but is also sometimes used by aromatherapists to help with disorders such as dermatitis. Useful for problem skins and a drop or two can be used in facial oils for helping acne. Juniper has a similar aroma to pine and blends well with resin, wood, herb, spice and citrus oils, notably galbanum, pine, cedarwood, clary sage and sandalwood.

LABDANUM (*Cistus ladaniferus*)

Source: A resin-gum from a small shrub. Native to the Mediterranean and Middle East.

Background: This attractive shrub produces beautiful creamy coloured flowers, inset with deep red. It is also known as Rock Rose as it produces such attractive flowers, although it is the leaves and twigs that contain the fragranced oils and not the flowers. The aromatic gum is produced by boiling the brown mass collected from its sticky leaves and stems. This antiseptic unguent was used by ancient civilisations to treat many different ailments, including wound healing, catarrh and dysentery. It was also burned as a powerful and purifying incense. A favourite ingredient for perfumers, labdanum acts as a natural fixative for many fine fragrances. Spain is now the largest producer of labdanum gum.

Actions: Antiseptic, anti-microbial, astringent, tonic.

Properties: Not commonly used in aromatherapy, but reputedly useful for helping to improve bronchial and respiratory conditions. May be added to essential oil blends for its aromatic aroma. Suits dry and mature skin types and can even be found in creams specifically formulated to help with psoriasis and eczema. The main identified chemical constituents of the essential oil are terpenes, acetophenone and other ketones.

Uses: An interesting and unusual addition to bath and massage oil blends, used mainly for its soft, subtle aroma. Acts as a natural fixative for other essential oils and blends well with lavender, pine, bergamot, clary sage and citrus oils.

LAVENDER (*Lavandula angustifolia*)

Source: Flower spikes from the herb. Native to Europe.

Background: From the Latin *lavare* meaning 'to bathe', lavender oil is one of the most versatile of all essential oils. The oil is contained in the tiny green pods that sit either side of its pale purple flowers. Used in fragrances and skin care for hundreds of years, lavender oil was the first English essential oil to be distilled commercially in the late 17th century. The oil is the main ingredient in lavender water, first created at about the same time. Lavender oil remains an important component of many fine fragrances and high-quality skin care treatments. The main producer of lavender oil is France, although this can be blended or adulterated before sale. As an example of this, France exports around 200 tonnes of 'lavender oil' and yet it grows only 40 tonnes! When buying for Liz Earle Cosmetics, our specialist will only buy the distilled essence immediately from the still to ensure its purity.

Good-quality oil is also produced in both Tasmania and Bulgaria. English lavender oil is also well known although it is produced on a much smaller scale, principally on farms in Norfolk. Lavender is not best-suited to British soil as it is not sufficiently sandy to allow the drainage required. The resulting British lavender oil tends to have a more camphorous odour. Some of the best scented lavender is grown above 1500 metres at high altitude in southern France.

Lavandin is an excellently scented oil that is extracted from hybrid lavender plants. It was created in the 1920s when the true lavender plant (*Lavandula officinalis*) was crossed with another pure variety called 'spike' lavender (*Lavandula latifolia*). The resulting plant is called *Lavandula hybrida*. Many aromatherapists turn their noses up at using lavandin, but it is a naturally extracted essential oil from a lavender plant. Many other essential oils are extracted from hybrid plants, for example peppermint or *Mentha piperita*, without any stigma. The problem has been more to do with the fact that lavandin essential oil has been confused with a more commonly used lavandin perfumery absolute. Pure lavandin essential oil has a better floral fragrance and a more intense 'lavender' aroma than *Lavandula officinalis*. As it is a hardier plant and easier to grow it is also usually less expensive.

Actions: Antiseptic, antibiotic, anti-viral, anti-fungal, balancing, fortifying, toning.

Properties: The most useful of all essential oils and a must-have for the first aid box. Excellent for treating infections and inflammatory disorders. Its gentle balancing action is reputed to be able to either calm or stimulate according to what is needed. However, clinical trials suggest that its action is more calming than stimulating. Researchers at Northumbria University, Newcastle, found that exposing volunteers to lavender essential oil vapours slowed their reaction times, reduced attention span and impaired their working memory – the part of the brain that puts facts 'on hold' before storing them in long-term memory. According to researcher Dr Mark Moss, 'Lavender seems to have a consistent sedative effect.' Lavender essential oil is also highly effective for treating burns when small quantities are applied topically. Also used by aromatherapists to help general infections, abrasions, colds, flu, stress, nausea, ulcers, acne, boils, rheumatism, sunburn, nervous tension and depression The main identified chemical constituents of both lavender and lavandin are linaly lacetate, linalool with coumarin, geraniol and limonene.

Uses: Use in very small quantities neat to heal burns. Dilute with wheatgerm oil or liquid vitamin E to reduce the appearance of scar tissue. Add a few drops to the bath for a fortifying effect. A firm, but gentle scalp, neck and shoulder massage with lavender oil can also help relieve tension headaches and migraine. Lavender oil can be burned or diffused in hospitals or sick rooms to promote an atmosphere of wellbeing. Suits most skin types except the very dry. An excellent addition to most massage blends and also for children. Blends well with most essential oils or may be used on its own.

LEMON (*Citrus limonum*)

Source: Rind from the fruit. Native to Europe.

Background: One of the simplest oils to extract from the oil glands on the fruit's outer peel, lemon oil is a traditional antiseptic and purifier. Associated with the hair and scalp, it is reputed to stimulate hair growth and will bleach hair blonde if applied and exposed to the sun. Most citrus oils have a limited shelf-life and should be used within about a year of purchase. Today, most modern lemon oil production is for the food and drink industry where it is widely used as a natural flavouring.

Actions: Antiseptic, antibiotic, anti-fungal, diuretic, stimulating.

Properties: Used to help stimulate the circulation and ward off infections. Useful for helping to lessen the severity of colds, sinusitis and sore throats, lemon oil may also be used by aromatherapists to help digestive disorders, gallstones, stress and anxiety. The main identified chemical constituents of the essential oil are limonene with pinene, citral, linalool and geraniol.

Uses: Add to massage oils to help improve blood circulation and skin tone. May be used neat in very small quantities as a local anti-septic. Useful for helping to clear blemished skin, it is also often added to massage blends to help tone flabby skin and improve the appear-ance of cellulite. Has a limited shelf-life so best kept cool and dark, and used within 12 months of opening. All expressed citrus oils can react strongly to sunlight and should not be used on the skin while sunbathing or before using a sunbed. There is no risk of photo-sensitivity with distilled citrus oils. Blends well with woody, resin, floral and spice oils, notably lavender, petitgrain, labdanum, neroli and ginger.

LEMON BALM (*Melissa officinalis*)

Source: Leaves from the herb. Native to Europe.

Background: Lemon balm is so-called because the leaves release a delicate lemon-like fragrance when rubbed with the fingers. Usually known as melissa, this oil is very different and much more expensive than lemon essential oil. Melissa thrives in Mediterranean countries and produces a highly fragrant oil that is popular for perfumes and aftershaves. Together with angelica extract, melissa was a key ingredient in 'balm water' made by Carmelite monks in medieval times. This highly prized fragrance was the world's first unisex scent and was worn by both noblemen and women. The local Mediterranean name for the herb was 'heart's delight' and infusions of the dried leaves were reputed to act as a tonic for heart-ache, both physical and romantic. Today, herbalists may use an infusion or extract from the leaves to treat tenseness, restlessness and general irritability. Numerous laboratory studies have shown lemon balm to have a sedative effect and also an anti-spasmodic effect on the bowel, but this is unlikely to apply to the pure essential oil. Melissa essential oil has been classified by some as a skin irritant, although some scientists dispute this and levels of up to 2 per cent have been found to be safe for use on the skin.

The name melissa comes from the Greek word for 'bee', as bees love the lemon balm flowers for making honey. Unfortunately, melissa oil wins a dubious prize for being one of the most commonly adulterated essential oils. One acre of land, cropped twice a year will yield just 1 kg of melissa essential oil, so it is no wonder that it is both rare and expensive. Pure melissa is quite commonly diluted with wintergreen, lemon, pine and citronella oils so always buy from a reputable source. Sometimes oils are labelled as a 'melissa blend' and combined with May chang (*Litsea cubeba*), Copahu balsam (*Copaifera officinalis*) and Clove bud (*Eugenia caryophyllus*).

Actions: Antiseptic, anti-viral, tonic, anti-depressant, sedative.

Properties: Can help treat nerves, over-exertion and stress. Useful to help treat digestive disorders and bacterial infections. Reputed to help slow the system, lower blood pressure and have an antispasmodic effect on overworked muscles. May also help lessen the severity of cold sores if applied in tiny quantities at the first sign of skin tingling. The main identified chemical constituents of the essential oil are geranial, neral, linalool and citronellal.

Uses: Add a few drops to a warm bath to help unwind and promote relaxation. May be included in massage blends specifically for use after exercise. Also useful added to massage blends for its rejuvenating tonic effects. Suits all skin types. Blends well with herb, spice, wood and resin essential oils.

MANDARIN (*Citrus nobilis*)

Source: Rind from the fruit. Native to Italy.

Background: Extracted from the tiny glands on the rind of mandarins, this fruit is an important crop in Italy, Brazil, Spain, Argentina and China. An inexpensive oil, it is an important ingredient for the perfume industry. Citrus essential oils should be used within about a year of purchase.

Actions: Antiseptic, fortifying, toning.

Properties: Used therapeutically by aromatherapists as a general tonic and natural tranquilliser. May help with insomnia, stress and nervous tension. Generally similar in its properties to orange oil. The main identified chemical constituent of the essential oil is limonene, with some linalool.

Uses: Add to a warm bath for an uplifting, toning effect. Add to massage oil blends to help boost the circulation and discourage water retention. Good for combination and problem skins. Mandarin is a citrus oil which, if expressed, can sensitise the skin when exposed to sunlight. Do not use on the skin while sunbathing or before using a sunbed or choose a distilled version. Blends well with spice and herb oils.

MARJORAM (*Origanum majorana*)

Source: Flowering tops and leaves from the herb. Native to Hungary.

Background: Also known as Sweet Marjoram, this versatile European herb produces a spicy oil with a warming action. In hot climates, the plant secretes a sweet, sticky resin from its stems which is popular with honey bees. Marjoram is probably best known for its culinary uses where it is associated as a poultry seasoning. It has a warm, spicy aroma, similar to cardamom and nutmeg.

Actions: Antiseptic, calming, sedative.

Properties: Used to help regulate the nervous system and may be useful in cases of insomnia. Induces drowsiness and in excess can have a mildly narcotic effect (to such an extent that it is reputed to lessen sexual ardour!). Used by aromatherapists to help with menstrual problems, menopausal disorders, anxiety and stress. Can help ease aches, sprains and intestinal cramps. The main identified chemical constituent of the essential oil is linalool, with some limonene.

Uses: Use a few drops in the bath before bedtime to promote a good night's sleep. Add to massage oils to help ease strained muscles and tired, aching limbs. Suits oily and combination complexions. Blends well with floral and citrus oils, notably lavender and bergamot.

MAY CHANG (*Litsea cubeba*)

Source: Fruits of the tree. Native to Asia.

Background: The Chinese may chang tree belongs to the laurel family (*Lauraceae*, like rosewood and cinnamon) and has long been revered for its fragrant flowers, fruits and leaves. However, its essential oil was not widely extracted from its small, pepper-like fruits until the 1950s. Its root and bark are traditional ingredients in Chinese herbal medicine. May chang is predominantly cultivated in Asia with most essential oil supplies coming from China, Japan and Taiwan. Traditionally, silkworms are fed on mulberry and may chang leaves although the oil can also be used as an insecticide. Its essential oil is produced by steam distillation of the fruit. May chang is a common fragrance ingredient in air fresheners and toiletries and is also a rich natural source for the antiseptic ingredient geramial citral, estimated to be as high as 75 per cent in the essential oil.

Actions: Antiseptic, disinfectant, digestive, tonic.

Properties: May chang has a similar aroma to lemongrass and is intensely lemony with a fresh, herby fragrance. However, it is more subtly scented than lemongrass, which can dominate a blend, and is an excellent addition to fragrance oils for the bath or massage. It is also used by aromatherapists to help treat oily and problem skins as well as for helping to combat digestive disorders. The main identified chemical constituents of the essential oil are geranial, citral, limonene, linalool and geraniol, and it is chemically similar in composition to lemongrass and melissa (lemon balm). Bafflingly described by some as a skin irritant (the sensitisation risk, due to its high citral level, is lessened by the presence of the limonene, linalool and geraniol), may chang is in fact a wonderful essential oil to use in blends.

Uses: A useful aromatic addition to bath and massage blends for the body. Best suits oily and combination skin types for facial massage and its antiseptic properties may be of benefit for acne conditions. May chang blends well with all citrus oils, rosemary, lavender and other florals. However, its aroma rapidly disappears, so is best used with a fixative oil such as galbanum or patchouli if you are intending to keep the blend for any length of time. May chang essential oil may increase photo-sensitivity so avoid using on the skin during sun exposure. The essential oil may also be a mild skin sensitiser in hot, humid conditions.

MELISSA (SEE LEMON BALM)

MYRRH (*Commiphora myrrha*)
Source: Bark and resin from the bush. Native to Somalia.

Background: First extracted more than 3000 years ago, myrrh comes from a small, thorny bush-like tree. Originally used by the Egyptians to embalm mummies and perfume linen. Egyptian women wore small pieces of cloth impregnated with myrrh oil around their necks and its fragrance was released by their body heat. The essential oil was one the three Magis' gifts to the infant Christ and one of the most popular perfumes of Ancient Greece was based on myrrh oil. Traditionally associated with the mouth, some 2000 years ago the physician Dioscorides stated that 'myrrh doth strengthen the teeth and ye gummies'. Pliny also recorded that the ingredients for a sore skin ointment called *susinum* consisted of cinnamon, saffron and myrrh. To increase the production of myrrh today, the collectors cut the tree bark to encourage the resin to ooze out. Some of the gum may fall to the ground where it picks up sand and grit, while other pieces may have to be peeled away from the tree. This method of collection produces myrrh of varying qualities and aromas.

Actions: Antiseptic, anti-inflammatory, cooling.

Properties: Useful for helping to improve chest complaints such as bronchitis and catarrh. Helps to heal burns and minor skin abrasions. Improves digestive disorders and is used in the treatment of fungal infections, including candidiasis. The main identified chemical constituents of the essential oil are sesquiterpenes, including heerabolene.

Uses: Popular in skincare oils to soothe inflamed skin, a few drops can be added to body massage oils to help tone the skin. Suits combination or oily complexions. Myrrh blends well with other resins, wood and heavily scented essential oils, including sandalwood, cypress and juniper berry. It also works well with citrus oils.

MYRTLE (*Myrtus communis*)

Source: Leaves and twigs from the tree. Native to North Africa.

Background: This attractive shrubby tree grows wild in many areas of the Mediterranean and its essential oil is produced mainly in Corsica and Spain. The plant is related to the aromatic eucalyptus and tea tree, as well as wax myrtle *Myrica cerifera* and bog myrtle *Myrica gale*. The latter two are not used in aromatherapy, as their oil is believed to be too toxic, although they have been used in herbal medicine. The myrtle bush is popular with gardeners as it is hardy, easy to grow and produces sweetly scented, frothy white flowers during the spring and summer.

Actions: Antiseptic, astringent, expectorant.

Properties: A pleasantly scented essential oil that has been used principally in the past for its fresh, herby aroma. Myrtle oil has been used in cough syrups for its gentle expectorant properties and is sometimes used to help treat coughs, colds and chest infections. The main identified chemical constituents of the essential oil are limonene, linalool, geraniol, eugenol, coumarin, myrtenol and nerol.

Uses: Myrtle is not a commonly used essential oil, which is a pity because it does have a delicious aroma. It best suits oily or combination skin types and is a useful addition to facial and massage oils. Blends well with floral, citrus and herb oils, notably neroli and orange.

NEROLI (*Citrus aurantium amara*)

Source: Flowers from the tree. Native to southern Europe.

Background: Also known as orange blossom or bitter orange flower oil, neroli is steam-distilled from the flowers of the bitter orange tree. Neroli is probably named after Princess Anne-Marie of Nerola, who used neroli oil in the 16th century to scent her gloves and bath water. Neroli has a distinctively soft, fruity aroma and remains an important ingredient in modern eau-de-colognes. It sits alongside rose, jasmine and ylang ylang as being one of the most important perfume ingredients today. Some of the best neroli oil comes from Morocco, Tunisia and Spain. It is one of the finest flower oils and, unfortunately, also one of the rarest and most expensive. The flowers must be processed as soon as they have been picked as they rapidly deteriorate. The neroli harvest can be dramatically affected by frost and in some years this can push its price up even higher. Recent harvests have been very poor due to changing weather conditions and prices have rocketed skywards. Genuine neroli essential oil is also increasingly rare and the average global crop is estimated at fewer than 500kg. The vast majority of 'neroli' fragrances use a synthetic copy. As neroli is not quite soluble in water significant amounts of the essential oil remain behind in the hydrolat during distillation. The resulting 'orange flower water' is highly prized for both its precious scent and skin caring attributes.

Actions: Antiseptic, antibiotic, uplifting.

Properties: One of my own all-time favourites, neroli warms and relaxes the body. Useful for helping to relieve anxiety and nervous tension. Reputed to help calm pre-exam or interview nerves and is sometimes recommended to help stage fright. Neroli is traditionally considered to be a very feminine oil and may help menopausal and hormonal disorders. The main identified chemical constituents of the essential oil are linalool, limonene and some farnesol, geraniol, jasmone and nerol (which gives neroli its very distinctive scent).

Uses: A few drops in a massage oil can help improve a sluggish circulation and perk up a tired complexion. Useful for blends to treat problem skins, neroli seems to benefit all skin types, even the sensitive. Creates a deliciously decadent and fortifying bath. Blends well with most oils, especially lavender, sandalwood, rose and rosemary.

PATCHOULI (*Pogostemon cablin*)
Source: Dried leaves from the herb. Native to Indonesia.

Background: Also known as *Pogostemon cablin*, the patchouli plant looks similar to lemon balm or mint and the highly scented oil glands are scattered over its labiate leaves. These produce a rich, claret-coloured oil with legendary skincare attributes. Originally used in the Far East and India as an aphrodisiac and household purifier. The first recorded use of patchouli oil in Europe was by the weavers of Paisley in Scotland who discovered that they could not compete with the Indian shawl exporters unless they impregnated their cloth with the same heady patchouli fragrance. Before the essential oil can be extracted, the leaves require crushing to break down their cell walls to release the aromatic compounds. This can be done in many ways, including blanching or scalding the leaves with hot water, but stacking or 'baling' the dried leaves before processing produces some of the most aromatic oil. Patchouli oil has a typically heavy, Eastern aroma and is an important ingredient in many spice-based perfumes where it is also used as a natural fixative. Recently classified as a mild photo-sensitiser, although there is little supporting evidence for this.

Actions: Antiseptic, stimulating, anti-fungal, fortifying.

Properties: A popular, multi-purpose oil reputed to be mildly aphrodisiac. Used by aromatherapists to help improve the circulation and soothe skin conditions. Can help treat fungal infections, acne and scalp disorders including dandruff. The main identified chemical constituents of the essential oil are sesquterpenes, patchoulene and azulene (a potent anti-inflammatory).

Uses: As it suits most complexions, patchouli oil is a useful addition to many skincare oils. May be diluted with wheatgerm oil or liquid vitamin E and applied to scar tissue or mild burns. Useful for toning the skin and it is a popular ingredient in treatments to help combat cellulite. Add to scalp oils to stimulate healthy hair growth. Releases an attractive, heady aroma when burned or diffused and a few drops turn bath time into a sensual treat. Blends well with floral, spice and citrus essential oils, especially sandalwood, bergamot, orange and neroli.

PEPPERMINT (*Mentha piperita*)

Source: The whole plant. Native to Europe.

Background: True peppermint essential oil is steam-distilled from the partially dried herb *Mentha piperita*, a hybrid from two other species of *Mentha*. Legend links its name to a mythological Greek nymph Mentha, whom the god Pluto found extremely alluring. Persephone, his jealous wife, chased Mentha away from Pluto and trod her into the ground, whereupon Pluto transformed her into a delightful herb. The peppermint variety is pungent, fresh-smelling oil that comes from the European herb named by the British botanist John Rea in 1700 for its peppery smell. China and India produce most of our peppermint oil, but European varieties have a more sought-after aroma. Peppermint leaves contain the compound menthol that contributes to its strong smell and feeling of coolness when rubbed on the skin. One rare variety called Mitcham Peppermint is produced in small quantities in the UK and contains unusually high levels of menthylesters, which give the oil a sweeter aroma and lessen its cooling action on the skin.

Peppermint essential oil is traditionally used in aftershaves and skin tonics for its invigorating action. Peppermint is also the most cultivated essential oil in the world, mainly for supplying the food, confectionery and toothpaste industries. Peppermint is also a well-known aid to digestion, for example, peppermint tea. Capsules of pure peppermint essential oil are also sold to help relieve indigestion, colic, nausea and irritable bowel syndrome – an example of how essential oils can safely be used internally.

Actions: Antiseptic, invigorating, anti-irritant, stimulating, refreshing.

Properties: Used to help lessen headaches, migraine and insomnia. Clears the head and encourages positive thinking. Has an antispasmodic action that is useful for relieving wind, heartburn, indigestion, nausea and colic. Unfortunately, peppermint is one of the most genetically modified herbs as high-quality, traditionally cultivated crops can only be cut once after two to three years' maturation. It is therefore worth seeking out organically grown peppermint oil as this will be GM-free. The main identified chemical constituents of the essential oil are menthol with menthone, limonene, cineole, pulegone and linalool.

Uses: Add to massage oils or facial spritzers for its invigorating and refreshing effect. Not the best choice for a bath oil (unless treating sunburn) as it makes the water feel cold against the skin. Suits oily and combination complexions best. Blends well with most herb, spice, wood and resin oils.

PETITGRAIN (*Citrus aurantium amara*)

Source: Leaves and twigs from the tree. Native to southern Europe.

Background: This woody-smelling oil is steam-distilled from the leaves of the bitter orange tree, traditionally grown in the warm, humid climates of southern France, Morocco and West Africa. The name petitgrain comes from the French word for 'little bit', referring to the tiny droplets of oil encapsulated in the leaves. The oil is also sometimes referred to as Petitgrain Bigarade oil, as *le bigaradier* is the French term for the bitter orange tree, *Citrus aurantium*, sub-species *amara*. In this context, 'bitter' is used to describe the aroma, which perfumers describe as a sort of dryness. This aroma comes from its high levels of terpenic compounds, which not only give the oil a dryer fragrance but also a fresh herby scent. Paraguay produces much of the best quality petitgrain oil from wild and semi-wild grown trees.

Actions: Antiseptic, calming, fortifying.

Properties: Used by aromatherapists to help aid an overburdened nervous system. Can help relieve anxiety and tension. Useful for insomnia and as a general aid to convalescence. Also used to help calm and balance the skin. The main identified chemical constituent of the essential oil is linalool, with some geraniol, limonene, dipentene and citral.

Uses: Add a few drops to a bath before bed time to promote a good night's sleep. Petitgrain releases off a warm, subtle aroma when burned or diffused. Suits dry, mature and sensitive skins. An excellent oil to add to massage blends for its fragrance as well as therapeutic properties and is often used as a less expensive alternative to neroli. Blends well with citrus, spice and herb oils (notably to help boost the aroma of neroli) orange and lavender.

PINE (*Pinus sylvestris*)

Source: Needles and wood from the tree. Native to America.

Background: One of the first essential oils documented by Dr Jean Valnet for its power to prevent and improve respiratory disorders, this variety of pine essential oil is produced from the heartwood and stumpwood from *Pinus sylvestris* and other *Pinus* species. Production takes place mostly in the USA, particularly in Florida and Maine, but many other *Pinus* oils are produced in the Far East. So-called pine oil is produced around the globe, but may in reality come from a by-product of the turpentine industry. These 'pine oils' may smell similar but posses none of pine oil's true therapeutic benefits. Pine essential oil may also be extracted from the leaves (needles) of several other varieties of pine tree, including *P. leucodermis, bor, nigra,* and *pumilo*. However, *Pinus pumilo* essential oil comes from the Dwarf Pine and is considered toxic, so should not be used in aromatherapy. Most aromatherapists seek to use *Pinus sylvestris* (Scotch Pine) as this is considered to be the best quality. Pine oil is associated with cleanliness and freshness and it is commonly added to medicated soaps and household cleaners. The essential oil possesses broad-spectrum anti-bacterial and anti-microbial properties.

Actions: Antiseptic, antibiotic, purifying, stimulating.

Properties: Useful for treating colds, 'flu, bronchitis and other respiratory infections. Strongly antiseptic, so useful for general infections and minor skin abrasions. Sometimes used by aromatherapists to help with bladder and kidney disorders and to improve the circulation. Studies show pine essential oil can also stimulate fibroblast activity within the skin, helping to increase epidermal cell turnover. The main identified chemical constituents of the essential oil are terpineol, estragole, fenchone and borneol.

Uses: Pine is a potent oil and so should be used sparingly. Use a few drops in a bowl of hot water as a steam inhalation. It may be burned or diffused to release a cleansing aroma. One or two drops in the bath during the winter months will help stave off infections and boost a sluggish circulation; however, greater quantities can irritate sensitive skins. Blends well with other wood oils, spice and citrus oils.

RAVENSARA (*Ravensara aromatica*)

Source: From the leaves. Native to Madagascar.

Background: Ravensara oil is distilled from the leaves of this ever-green Laurel-style tree which grows wild around the Indian Ocean and is also cultivated in France. Used in India as an effective natural remedy against plague and other highly acute infectious diseases. Not much is documented about ravensara although it has an almost mythical status as a supremely healing essential oil. However, little safety or toxicological data has been established with its use.

Actions: Antiseptic, anti-bacterial, anti-viral, anti-microbial, anti-fungal, tonic.

Properties: An extraordinary and unusual essential oil that is highly prized by many naturopaths and aromatherapists for its ther-apeutic properties. Ravensara essential oil is extremely potent – 20 times more powerful than tea tree oil – yet it is gentle on the skin and has a pleasantly mild scent. Its slightly medicinal, eucalyptus-like aroma is subtly sweet with a fruity, citrus top-note. Ravensara is reputed to help treat shingles by both treating the infection and helping to clear the skin. Also believed to help strengthen the immune system. The main identified chemical constituents of the essential oil are estragole, found in many antiseptics, together with pinene, caryophyllene and terpineol. True ravensara (not to be confused with ravinsara from Madagascan camphor which has a similarly high linalool content) contains less than 5 per cent cineol.

Uses: May be used topically on the skin, either neat in tiny quan-tities or blended into massage oil. Useful for burning or diffusing, or using as compresses for damaged skin and soft tissue injuries.

ROSE (*Rosa damascena*)

Source: Flower petals. Native to the Middle East.

Background: Also known as Rose Bulgar, Otto of Rose or Attar of Roses, this fragrant oil comes from ruby-red damascena roses. Legend has it that the damask rose was created from a single drop of sweat falling from the prophet Mohammed's brow. The flower later gave its name to the city of Sanascus and the heavy silk fabric that was originally woven there. The essential oil is now principally cultivated in the valley of Kazenlik in Bulgaria. As the sun rises over the Balkan foothills the precious oil content of the roses drops dramatically due to evaporation. The blooms that have flowered must therefore be picked very early in the morning. Genuine Rose Otto is distinguished by its yellow-greenish colour and at low temperatures has a semi-solid, almost crystalline texture. Pure rose oil contains over 500 different chemical constituents and so far has proved impossible for the cosmetic chemists to copy exactly. We do know that the petals contain bioflavonoids and tannins as major components which have antiseptic, stimulatory and astringent actions respectively. Rose remains one of the most important perfume ingredients and is found in many fine fragrances. Rose oil is one of Nature's most versatile extracts and is reported to have a specific healing action on the liver. In traditional Indian medicine rose is used for sore throats and tonsilitis, headaches and skin disorders. It is also mixed with sesame oil to produce a nourishing hair oil known as Gul-Roghan.

Actions: Antiseptic, uplifting, nourishing, soothing.

Properties: Traditionally associated with soothing dry, mature skins. Used by aromatherapists to help treat mild depression and fatigue. Can help PMS and symptoms of the menopause. As it takes around 40,000 individual blooms to make a single ounce of rose oil, 67 roses go into every drop! No wonder pure rose oil is so very expensive. The main identified chemical constituents of the essential oil are citronellol and geraniol, with some citral, eugenol, linalool, farnesol and other constituents.

Uses: A luxury oil to be used sparingly in facial massage blends or added in tiny quantities to a bath. A wonderful oil for sensitive skins and small children. Also makes a fabulously pampering skin treatment for the body. Suits dry, mature and sensitive complexions. Blends well with other delicate flower oils (especially jasmine) and soft woods or resins such as sandalwood and frankincense.

ROSE ABSOLUTE (*Rosa centifolia*)

Source: Flower petals. Native to South-East Asia.

Background: Rose absolute is widely used in aromatherapy and although it is not a true essential oil it is highly regarded for its fabulous, pure aroma. Rose absolute is produced by solvent extraction from the pale pink *centifolia* or *Rose de Mai*. The *centifolia* variety bears few oil-producing glands and is used more for its fragrance than any other therapeutic purpose. Following solvent extraction, rose absolute is distilled with alcohol and there is a feeling amongst many professionals that traces of the chemical solvent may be carried through to the end product. When choosing rose absolute it is important to know the source of the oil and to know that it has been tested for its purity. Pure rose absolute is highly concentrated and expensive. As a result, what is most commonly sold as rose essential oil is more likely to be a dilution of the absolute. Common additives include rosewood and rose-scented geranium, as these intensify the rose aroma. Rose absolute is a very important element in perfume and the *centifolia* roses have been cultivated by perfumiers in Grasse since the 16th century. Rose absolute was first distilled in Persia and remains an important Middle Eastern flavouring. It is most commonly used in sweetmeats such as Turkish delight.

Action: Antiseptic, uplifting fragrance.

Properties: The main benefits from rose absolute come from its fabulous smell and antiseptic properties. It is used in high-quality skincare for its gently toning and reviving properties. The main identified chemical constituents of the essential oil are citronellol and geraniol, with some citral, eugenol, linalool and farnesol.

Uses: As for rose oil. Also wonderful as a natural skin scent when diluted with a light, neutral carrier oil. Blends well with other delicate flower oils (especially jasmine) and soft woods or resins such as sandalwood and frankincense.

ROSEMARY (*Rosmarinus officinalis*)

Source: Flowering tops and twigs from the herb. Native to Spain.

Background: One of the oldest essential oils, rosemary belongs to the *Labiate* plant family, among which are many perfumed botanicals. The oil itself is stored in tiny oil glands just beneath the leaf's long smooth surface. The aroma is easily released when the leaves are rubbed between the fingers. Regarded as a sacred herb by the Ancient Greeks and Romans who often used it in ceremonial rituals. Traditionally associated with the head, the 17th-century English herbalist Culpeper prescribed two or three drops of oil rubbed onto the temples to help relieve headaches. Rosemary oil was also the base for the world's first commercially produced perfume called Hungary water, formulated in 1370.

The most famous literary reference is from Shakespeare's *Hamlet* when Ophelia declares, 'There's rosemary, that's for remembrance: pray, love, remember.' Recent studies have confirmed that rosemary essential oil can indeed aid memory as well as increasing attention and lifting mood. Researchers at Northumbria University, Newcastle, found that volunteers who sat in a booth filled with rosemary oil vapour were able to more quickly memorise a list of words and recall more of them after 30 minutes than a control group without the rosemary vapour. The essential oil seemed to enhance long-term memory by around 15 per cent and to have a stimulating affect on mood. Rosemary grows wild in many Mediterranean countries and good quality wild-grown essential oil can be found in France, Spain and Corsica.

Actions: Stimulating, antiseptic, invigorating, diuretic.

Properties: An excellent all-round tonic. Helps combat water retention and may help to improve cellulite. Useful for helping to relieve sprains and aching limbs, including arthritis. Used by aromatherapists to help relieve headaches, dandruff and even to combat hair loss. Has mild anti-spasmodic properties and may help to relieve coughs. Studies show rosemary essential oil can also stimulate fibroblast activity within the skin, helping to increase epidermal cell turnover. The main identified chemical constituents of the essential oil are limonene, pinene, camphor, cineole and borneol.

Uses: Use sparingly in massage oils or add a few drops to the bath as a potent pick-me-up. Can be used to help tone the skin and help the appearance of cellulite. Best suited to problem skins and oilier complexions. Blends well with spice, herb and citrus oils, notably lavender, lemon, thyme, pine, petitgrain and labdanum.

ROSEWOOD (*Aniba rosaeodora*)

Source: Wood chips from the tree. Native to Brazil.

Background: Also known as Brazilian Bois de Rose. Produced from the bark of the South American *Aniba rosaeodora* tree that belongs to the laurel family, so named for its lightly rose-scented wood. The tree is a medium-sized, tropical, wild-growing ever-green from the Amazon rainforest basin. Used as a less expensive alternative to rose petal oils, rosewood may have fewer therapeutic benefits than pure rose oil, but it does have a deliciously warm, sweet aroma. Although less costly than rose oil, pure rosewood is sometimes adulterated with synthetic linalool. Environmentalists should be especially aware that some countries may not be enforc-ing the Convention on International Trade in Endangered Species (CITES) laws when it comes to rosewood, so always buy from a supplier who fully respects this to help preserve its availability for the future. The main supplies come from the rapidly diminishing rainforests of Brazil, where the essential oil production (from steam-distilled wood chips) is actually a by-product of the lumbar industry. Replanting schemes have already been implemented but young trees are struggling in the impoverished soils. Even if these schemes succeed it will take about 30 years for the trees to become mature enough to produce a commercially viable amount of essen-tial oil. In the meantime, rosewood oil can be distilled from the leaves of the growing trees, but it will have different properties to the oil produced from the bark.

An increasingly popular alternative to rosewood oil is ho wood, produced from the camphor tree *Cinnamomum camphora*. This is increasingly farmed in properly managed plantations in Formosa, China and Japan. A rose-scented essential oil may be steam distilled from both the bark and wood (ho wood oil) or the leaves (ho leaf oil).

Actions: Antiseptic, antibacterial, toning.

Properties: Used by aromatherapists to help relieve headaches. A good anti-depressant and useful tonic to improve mood and ward off general malaise. The main identified chemical constituents of the essential oil are linalool with cineole, limonene and geraniol.

Uses: A good all-purpose essential oil that can be used in place of real rose oil for its lovely fragrance. Useful in body massage blends and also in the bath as a pick-me-up. Blends well with many oils, including the florals such as geranium and citrus oils.

SAGE (*Salvia officinalis*)

Source: Flowering tops from the herb. Native to Europe.

Background: A sacred herb from the Ancient world, sage has a distinct and strongly pungent aroma. It is classified as being different botanically to clary sage and it has a very different aroma. Sage has many medicinal properties and is believed to take its botanical name from the Latin word *salvia*, meaning salvation. Sage will grow in most parts of Britain, although our supplies of the oil tend to come from Mediterranean countries, Dalmatian sage being the most well known. Sage is most commonly used as a culinary herb and is an important ingredient for vermouth and other alcoholic bitters. It is also an important ingredient in Chinese herbal medicine; however, due to its high thujone content, it is regarded as both toxic and skin irritating in large quantities and should be used with care.

Actions: Antiseptic, anti-fungal, stimulating, healing, toning.

Properties: A useful regulator of the central nervous system. Aromatherapists may use sage to treat depression, mild menstrual and digestive disorders. Useful against catarrh, bronchitis and other chest conditions. A strongly antiseptic herb with good antioxidant properties. Sore throats may be successfully treated with a gargle made with a herbal infusion of dried sage. The main identified chemical constituents of the essential oil are camphor, limonene and cineole.

Uses: A powerful oil which can overstimulate. Best used under the guidance of a well-qualified aromatherapist. Blends well with citrus and other herb oils, notably lavender, rosemary, orange and neroli.

SANDALWOOD (*Santalum album*)

Source: Bark and wood chippings from the tree. Native to India.

Background: A traditional Indian extract that dates back more than 4000 years, this oil comes from a parasitic tree that grows by attaching its roots to others. Although the tree grows to a height of 20–30 feet, only the inner wood, known as the 'heart wood', is used to extract the essential oil. Sandalwood has a rich, woody aroma and is burned by Hindus in temples and at all their religious occasions. Hindu spiritual leaders paint their foreheads with sandalwood paste as a symbol of purity. Sandalwood comes from one of the slowest-growing trees and it takes around 40 years before the essential oil can be extracted. The wood itself is popular for both building construction and for making furniture as it resists attack from pest, notably woodworm. Sandalwood oil is frequently diluted or adulterated before sale and so it is important to buy it from a reputable supplier. Indonesia is now also producing sandalwood essential oil but it is not as highly regarded. Sandalwood is increasingly rare and may become an endangered species. The Indian government has ordered that for every tree felled, two more must be planted, so check to make sure your supplier buys from a sustainable source.

Actions: Antiseptic, anti-irritant, mild analgesic, a reputed aphrodisiac.

Properties: Sandalwood oil has a high natural alcohol content so it is strongly antiseptic. A versatile and gentle oil with a subtle aroma that helps instil a sense of calm and wellbeing. Traditionally used as masculine oil, sandalwood has been used in natural medicine to help treat impotence. Australian sandalwood oil is also used in Aboriginal medicine as a treatment for urinary tract infections. Studies show sandalwood essential oil can also stimulate fibroblast activity within the skin, helping to increase epidermal cell turnover. The main identified chemical constituent of the essential oil is santenone alcohol.

Uses: A few drops in a warm bath make a useful tension-relieving pick-me-up. May be added to massage blends to help improve sore, bruised skin conditions. Suits difficult complexions and is useful in facial oil blends for many disorders, including flaking skin and acne. Blends well with spice, resin, citrus and floral oils, notably rose, lavender and bergamot.

SWEET ORANGE (*Citrus aurantium dulcis*)

Source: Peel of the fruit. Native to the Far East.

Background: Sweet orange oil was originally introduced to Europe from the Orient and the fruits from the orange tree were probably the legendary 'golden apples' in the Garden of Hesperides. This mythological garden contained fruits prized by the goddess Hera that were guarded by both the Hesperides, or the Daughters of Evening nymphs, and a multi-headed dragon named Ladon. One of Heracles famous 12 'labours' was to retrieve some of these so-called apples. An early documented therapeutic use of the orange is from the Ancient Roman era, when orange flower water was drunk to reduce hangovers. Today, oranges are principally grown in Brazil, the USA and the Mediterranean, with most of the essential oil being extracted in South America. The essential oil is a common byproduct of the huge orange juice industries so it is relatively inexpensive. However, as the orange crops tend to be sprayed with several fungicides and herbicides, which remain on the skin, it is worth choosing organic versions. This essential oil is also known as sweet orange oil.

Actions: Antiseptic, anti-inflammatory, anti-bacterial, uplifting, tonic.

Properties: Aromatherapists will often use orange oil to help improve mood and digestive disorders. It is an excellent tonic and helps to uplift and refresh the body. Orange oil is a natural anti-bacterial agent and is useful for its de-greasing and cleansing properties. Some environmentally friendly household cleaning products include orange oil for this reason. The main identified chemical constituents of the essential oil are limonene (around 95 per cent), small amounts of linalool and citral, and (in some cases) bergaptene.

Uses: A few drops added to a warm bath or mixed into a massage blend will give a reviving and toning effect. Pure, expressed orange essential oil can react mildly to sunlight and should not be used on the skin while sunbathing or before using a sunbed. The risk of such photo-sensitivity is much less likely with distilled orange oil. Orange essential oil has a limited shelf-life so is best kept cool and dark, and used within 12 months of opening. Blends well with other citrus oils, woody aromas, florals and resins.

TEA TREE (*Melaleuca alternifolia*)

Source: Leaves and twigs from the tree. Native to Australia.

Background: This interesting oil comes from the bark of a common Australian tree that is extremely resistant to disease. There are many different types of *Melaleuca*, the *alternifolia* being one of the smaller species. Tea trees have amazing powers of recuperation and if chopped down will quickly grow again from their original stump. The essential oil is highly renowned for its anti-viral and anti-fungal properties. Originally used in Aboriginal medicine, tea tree oil is increasingly used by conventional medics to treat skin disorders and fungal infections including candidiasis (thrush) and ringworm. Tea tree oil is about five times more effective at killing germs and bacteria than household disinfectant, while being kinder to the skin. Niaouli essential oil belongs to the tea tree oil family (it is extracted from *Melaleuca quinquenervia* and has a slightly sweeter, less sharp aroma than classic tea tree oil).

Actions: Antiseptic, antibiotic, anti-viral, anti-fungal.

Properties: Remarkably active against all three kinds of infectious organisms: bacterial, fungal and viral. Has even been reported effective against 100 different strains of methicillin- (or multiple-) resistant *Staphylococcus aureus* (MRSA), an increasingly common and very dangerous bacterium that is resistant to many antibiotics, which are responsible for outbreaks of infection in hospitals. As there have been cases of bugs that show resistance even to vancomycin – an antibiotic traditionally regarded as the 'last line of defence' – the properties of tea tree oil could be especially important. One study found that in 25 people with an MRSA infection, topical treatment with tea tree essential oil eradicated the infection after six weeks of treatment. Another study found that a dilution of just 2.5 per cent tea tree essential oil was more effective against MRSA than a conventional antiseptic. Tea tree oil may also be helpful when used in massage blends to ward off less dangerous coughs, colds and flu. It is used to treat skin disorders including cold sores, warts and burns, and trials by Australian dermatologists have shown it to be as effective at treating acne as orthodox treatment using benzoyl peroxide, but with fewer side-effects. The main identified chemical constituent of the essential oil is terpin-4-ol, with some linalool.

Uses: Use neat in very small amounts to treat spots, burns and insect bites. Add a small quantity to scalp oils to help clear dandruff and scalp disorders. A few drops in the bath is reputed to help combat the effects of shock, as well as being highly cleansing and purifying for the skin. Blends well with citrus, tree, herb and floral oils, especially lavender, rosemary and pine. Preferably, buy bottles with a use-by date and use within 12 months as old tea tree oil can cause skin sensitisation.

THYME (*Thymus vulgaris*)

Source: Flowering tops from the herb. Native to Europe.

Background: A medicinal herb known to the ancient world that is now used in herbal medicine throughout the world. Was commonly burnt as a household disinfectant to ward off rodents and get rid of fleas. Sprigs of fresh thyme can be hung in wardrobes instead of mothballs. The essential oil possesses broad-spectrum anti-bacterial and anti-microbial properties. Thymol is its principal active constituent and it is a powerful antiseptic that must be used sparingly and with caution, although, interestingly, studies by American researchers have also shown thyme essential oil to have good anti-irritant properties. Its antiseptic properties can be found in many pharmaceutical products, including mouthwash, cough medicine, lozenges and toothpaste. Thyme oil that has been steam-distilled from the flowers only has a sweeter aroma than that distilled from the flowering tops and leaves. Lemon thyme and white thyme are considered to be the safest varieties to use on the skin. Red thyme should be avoided as it contains higher levels of powerful phenols (carvacrol and thymol), as should *Thymus capitus* or Spanish oregano.

Actions: Antiseptic, antibiotic, anti-fungal, anti-viral, stimulating.

Properties: Used by aromatherapists as a general tonic to relieve fatigue and anxiety. Stimulates the circulation and reputed to encourage the elimination of toxins. Reported to be a uterine stimulant that should be avoided during pregnancy. Highly anti-bacterial as well as strongly antioxidant, researchers at the Agricultural College in Aberdeen have found that thyme oil can help strengthen the immune system. Useful for tired, aching limbs and for using in tiny quantities to help treat a wide range of infections. The main identified chemical constituents of the essential oil are thymol and carvacrol (also geraniol and linalool, depending on plant variety).

Uses: An extremely potent oil that should be used under the guidance of an aromatherapist. A skin irritant in high concentrations, although a couple of drops well-diluted in a carrier oil can usefully be applied to wounds or rubbed across the throat to help infected or swollen glands. A powerful oil that will dominate other essential oils in a blend.

VETIVER (*Vetiveria zizanioides*)

Source: Dried roots from the grass. Native to India.

Background: Although native to India, this tall perennial grass is now grown in many volcanic areas as its extensive network of roots helps to protect the soil from erosion during the torrential tropical rains. In India it is particularly grown on the plains and lower hills, around the river banks and rich marshy soils of Kerala. The essential oil is steam-distilled from the grass's roots that have been washed, chopped and soaked in water prior to distilling. It has a fresh 'green' fragrance, sometimes likened to potato peelings, but actually much more attractive than this. Vetiver, or its fragrant component vetiverol, is widely used in many perfumes and aftershaves. The most sought after vetiver essential oil comes from Haiti, Reunion and the Belgian Congo.

Actions: Antiseptic, calming, soothing.

Properties: This sweet-smelling oil is used by aromatherapists to help reduce nervous tension and promote relaxation. Used in massage as a muscle relaxant. In skin care the oil is used to help heal skin blemishes as well as for its deliciously fresh, herby aroma. The main identified chemical constituents of the essential oil are

Hyssop
Juniper
Marjoram
Patchouli
Peppermint
Sage
Thyme
Vetiver

RESIN SCENTS

Benzoin
Frankincense
Galbanum
Myrrh

SPICE SCENTS

Black Pepper
Cardamom
Coriander
Ginger
Ravensara

WOOD SCENTS

Cajuput
Camphor
Cedarwood
Cypress
Eucalyptus
Pine
Sandalwood
Tea tree

Golden rules

Although all essential oils look much the same, their chemical content can vary considerably. As it is virtually impossible to tell exactly what is in the bottle, you will need to rely heavily on the integrity of the producers. As a general guide, you mostly get what you pay for and the most expensive oils are usually worth the extra cost. Serious aromatherapists usually prefer to buy most of their essential oils from specialists accredited by the International Federation of Aromatherapists (see Useful Resources, p.208). If you do buy essential oils from the high street, always read the label first. Those called 'fragrance oils', 'aromatic oils' or 'aromatherapy oils' are not essential oils at all, but inferior dilutions. They may contain all kinds of unwanted extras including synthetic perfumes and preservatives. Good quality essential oils should always be labelled with both their botanical name (in Latin, to be sure of the correct species) and their country of origin.

ORGANIC OILS

The answer to the question 'Should I buy organic essential oils?' is long-winded but important and it pays to have a working knowledge of ethno-botany, which includes the folklore and traditional uses of plants. Many essential oils are now labelled as 'organic' and although this is often an advantage, it is not a requirement in all cases. Disease-resistant trees such as frankincense, cypress and many other plants grown in developing countries where chemical sprays and fertilisers are not in general use are frequently organic, whether labelled so or not. Some suppliers charge inflated prices for 'organic' oil when it is invariably organic anyway. Ylang ylang is one example of an exotic oil that is not produced with chemical sprays or fertilisers. In addition, many small producers cannot afford to pay the registration fees charged by the organic certification organisations – yet their crops may be 100 per cent organically produced by traditional farming methods. After all, it is the method – and not the piece of paper – that makes any product organic. Organic jasmine or rose absolutes do not exist, as absolutes are extracted using solvents that are prohibited for any oil that carries official organic status.

'Wild-grown' or 'wild-crafted' are other terms that you may see on a label. These should mean that the oil has been naturally produced, often to organic standards, but that it does not have official organic certification. They are often a good choice, but bear in mind that some 'wild grown' producers have little respect for the environment and may be over-harvesting until no plants remain. Overall, the best option is to choose oils produced from organically cultivated or sustainably wild-grown plants.

SAFETY MEASURES

Bear in mind that essential oils are always highly concentrated and should be treated with care. They must be stored with tightly closed screw-cap lids (not corks) out of the reach of children. The edge of the bath is not an ideal place to keep pure essential oils ... For safety reasons, always buy essential oils that are fitted with an individual dropper stopper. This will enable you to measure the correct number of drops more accurately and will also reduce any chance of swallowing by an inquisitive child. If an essential oil is accidentally swallowed, drink as much water as possible and seek immediate medical attention. Try to avoid getting essential oils in the eyes or applying to mucous membranes such as the lips (except, as mentioned below, in the case of cold sores). If essential oils do come into contact with the eyes, some aromatherapists prefer to rinse them out with a pure vegetable oil, such as grapeseed or purified olive oil, which may absorb any residue of essential oil more effectively than water. Otherwise, eyes should be rinsed immediately and thoroughly with plenty of cool water. Don't forget that some essential oils are also highly flammable.

Generally speaking, essential oils should not be used neat on the skin. There are a few exceptions, such as lavender, which can be very helpful for helping to heal small burns and abrasions. Similarly, tiny dots of tea tree, ravensara and pine are useful natural antiseptics, while a dab of pure melissa (lemon balm) can help lessen the severity of cold sores if applied at first sign of tingling. If any redness, itching or irritation on the skin occurs, stop using the essential oil and apply a bland vegetable oil, such as purified olive oil, removing it with a muslin cloth or flannel. This will dilute any remaining residues on the skin and should be repeated several times until the skin is calm. This method of removing essential oils from the skin is much more effective than rinsing with water, which may further aggravate the problem. Obviously, all skins can react differently to any substance that is applied to them; however, very sensitive skins can react to the essential oils bay, basil, birch, cajuput, cassia, cedar leaf, cinnamon leaf, clove bud, fennel (sweet), lemon, lemongrass, peppermint, pine, tea tree and thyme. In addition, pure bergamot and some citrus oils can make the skin more sensitive to the sun's ultraviolet rays and should be avoided during sun (or sun-bed) exposure.

The best precaution when using any essential oils for the first time, or for those with sensitive skins, is always to do a small skin patch test first. This means applying a small amount of the essential oil, diluted in a blend if this is how you will be using it, to an area of fine skin, such as the inner arm. Leave for 24 hours and repeat two or three times for the most conclusive results. This is especially important if you are an 'allergic-type' – for example, if you have any history of asthma, eczema, allergic rhinitis or food sensitivities. Even if you do experience an adverse reaction, it could be worth repeating the patch test with a different brand, as an adulterant in the oil may be the cause of the problem and not the actual oil itself. A few essential oils, especially those of the citrus, pine and tea tree families, can develop skin sensitising chemicals with age. It is best not to use these varieties on the skin within six months of opening (thereafter they can be used for burning or diffusing). Keeping oils in a small, well-labelled box at the top of the fridge will also help prolong their shelf-life. When buying carrier or essential oils, choose a supplier with a frequent stock turnover and avoid old looking bottles with dusty lids! The preferred option is a bottle carrying a date stamp.

To preserve the potency of an essential oil blend it is important to store it in the right conditions. All oils should be kept in metal, amber or tinted glass bottles to protect them from spoilage caused by light. Essential oils should not be stored in plastic containers as they can dissolve chemicals within the plastic, which ruin the purity of the oil. Remember, oils are affected by oxygen in the air each time they are opened so buy them in small quantities and always replace the lids after use. You will find that essential oils last longer if kept in a cool place, such as in a box at the top of the fridge. If this is not possible, make sure the room temperature where they are kept does not exceed 15°C (79°F), so store in a cool cupboard away from any radiators or sunny windows.

Cautionary tales

Probably the most cause for concern for aromatherapy aficionados is how to get what we think we're getting when we buy essential oils. Making sure that the bottle labelled 'pure lavender essential oil' does indeed contain pure lavender oil and nothing else is a very tricky and complex business. It's impossible to tell exactly what is in a bottle of essential oil without using sophisticated analytical equipment, so a great deal of trust is involved. It's worth buying essential oils from suppliers who test each batch of oil as it arrives in their warehouse and who are able to trace their sources each step of the way, from harvesting in the field to filling the final bottle.

Many essential oil wholesalers are equipped with a Gas-Liquid spectrometer (GLS) or a Gas-Liquid Chromatographer (GLC). These useful items of laboratory equipment are helpful for detecting deliberate essential oil fraud or errors in labelling. They work by producing a printed graph showing the peaks and troughs that relate to various compounds. This enables a technician literally to 'read' the contents of an anonymous bottle to see what it contains. Samples of an essential oil can easily be tested to see whether the GLS or GLC machine produces a print-out that matches its chemical fingerprint. The operator should ensure that each print-out is scanned at various frequencies, as some can hide the inclusion of compounds such as preservatives. Reputable essential oil suppliers will test all their oils on arrival from their source, allowing variations for each constituent within the oil to account for differences in climate, soil quality and time of crop harvest.

Having selected your essential oils, correct storage conditions are also vital, as all essential oils need to be kept cool and dark for maximum shelf life. As with fine vintage wines, some essential oils can actually improve over time. For example, Aromatrading keep oils such as lavender for two years to allow the depth of fragrance to develop fully and they then re-test the essential oil before bottling. Finally, a good benchmark is often the price. Good quality essential oils are, without any doubt, always more expensive to produce than poor quality ones.

TOXICITY CONTROVERSIES

The issue of toxicity and essential oils is complicated and unclear. It is also an issue at the heart of an ongoing debate between some scientists, medical researchers and those in the aromatherapy business. The problem is that there are very few undisputed facts on the subject and even less in the way of credible medical research involving properly controlled clinical trials. Much that has been written over the years about the safety, or otherwise, of essential oils has evolved from mythical folklore. Originally, the plants that were documented for medicinal use as soluble extracts were either drunk or taken internally as herbal medicines. These extracts obviously have very different effects within the body than the distilled aromatic essential oils that are well-diluted before being applied topically on the skin. Unfortunately, many of the properties, benefits and side-effects recorded for these plants that were originally noted after internal use are now mistakenly linked to the essential oils. Any reviewer of aromatherapy textbooks can confirm that much of what is written is simply repeated from book to book to book, and it can be hard, if not impossible, to find the original source to investigate further. The same can be said of aromatherapy and essential oil web-sites, many of which repeat erroneous folk-lore and legend instead of proven facts.

The fact is that most essential oils are completely safe to use within the guidelines already mentioned. The oils most commonly reported to be highly toxic are, fortunately, not commonly available and so are easy to avoid. These include bitter almond, mugwort, sassafras (which contains safrol, banned under EU law in the levels found in the essential oil), rue, tansy, thuja, wintergreen and wormwood. A few other essential oils are also often deemed to be unsafe for home use and recommended only for use under the guidance of a qualified practitioner. These include clove, cinnamon, sage and thyme. However, it is worth noting that each of these oils is widely eaten in foods, on a daily basis in some cultures. So, the risk of occasionally rubbing a few drops onto the skin – a sophisticated organ designed to be the body's most highly effective barrier – must be so low as to be negligible. Some time-honoured pharmaceutical skin products are actually based on very high concentrations of potentially sensitising essential oils. For example, Tiger Balm, sold the world over as a muscle rub, consists of 60 per cent pure essential oils, including cassia, clove and camphor, yet no one suggests it is unsafe to use (even during pregnancy). When discussing the risk of using essential oils, it is important to put any potential problems into proper perspective.

The following essential oils are on the 'caution' list issued by the International Federation of Aromatherapists. This is because they may present risks of toxicity, skin irritation and/or skin sensitisation. None of these essential oils is commonly available for home use.

Almond (bitter)	*Prunus amygdalus*
Boldo leaf	*Peumus boldus*
Calamus	*Acorus calamus*
Camphor (brown oil)	*Cinnamomum camphora*
Camphor (yellow oil)	*Cinnamomum camphora*
Cassia	*Cinnamomum cassia*
Cinnamon (bark)	*Cinnamomum zeylanicum*
Costus	*Saussurea lappa*
Elecampane	*Inula helenium*
Fennel (bitter)	*Foeniculum vulgare*
Horseradish	*Armoracia rusticana*
Jaborandi (leaf)	*Pilocarpus jaborandi*

Mugwort	*Artemisia vulgaris*
Mustard	*Brassica nigra*
Pine (dwarf)	*Pinus mugo*
Rue	*Ruta graveolens*
Sassafras	*Sassafras albidum*
Sassafras (Brazilian)	*Octea cymbarum*
Savine	*Juniperus sabina*
Southernwood	*Artemisia abrotanum*
Tansy	*Tanacetum vulgare*
Thuja (cedarleaf)	*Thuja occidentalis*
Thuja (Western red/Washington)	*Thuja plicata*
Wintergreen	*Gaultheria procumbens*
Wormseed	*Chenopodium anthelminticum*
Wormwood	*Artemisia absinthium*

The legislation that covers the sale of essential oils is complicated. Essential oils do not have their own legal category and so, depending on their use, may come under the various governing laws for foods, cosmetics or medicines. For the latest on toxicity issues and legislation, see Useful Resources, p.208.

Essential oils and epilepsy

Although there is no sound scientific evidence for any essential oils causing epilepsy, it is widely reported in aromatherapy textbooks that oils containing high levels of ketones have been linked to triggering epilepsy. Essential oils that include higher than average levels of ketones amongst their chemical constituents include those in the 'danger' group above, together with hyssop, pennyroyal and crested lavender (*Lavandula stoechas* – not to be confused with the traditionally used varieties). Essential oils containing moderate levels of ketones include sage, spike lavender (*Lavandula latifolia*) – again not to be confused with the traditionally used varieties and camphor. Essential oils with a low ketone content include yarrow, rosemary, peppermint, eucalyptus and cedar wood. While there is no proof that these oils present any danger to epileptics, it is known that powerful aromas can trigger a seizure. Therefore, it would be sensible for all epileptics to avoid strong smells of all kinds, including perfumes. On the positive side, a relaxing aromatherapy massage has been found to be very soothing for those with epilepsy and can substantially reduce the incidence of attacks.

Essential oils and high blood pressure

Over the years, a few highly aromatic essential oils have been linked to causing disturbances with either high or low blood pressure. These oils include those similarly listed for epilepsy – notably hyssop, rosemary, sage and thyme. However, despite lengthy research I have not found any medical evidence or details of any clinical trials that supports this claim. Some researchers argue that a relaxing aromatherapy massage is likely to help balance the blood pressure and that this would be more likely to lower high blood pressure that has been raised by stress.

Essential oils and pregnancy

It is frequently said that essential oils should also be used with care during pregnancy as they have been shown to enter the bloodstream via inhalation and could, potentially, cross the placental barrier. It is impossible to be sure of the effect, if any, that essential oils might have on a developing baby. However, do remember that most of us will eat far more essential oils than we'll ever absorb through the skin! These will include essential oils from citrus peel (marmalade, fruit cake, etc.), herb teas, and culinary herbs such as rosemary, mint and basil, to name but a few. Unfortunately, much misinformation exists on the subject of essential oil safety during pregnancy. However, the fear is more legal than medical and is fuelled by the risk of expensive litigation rather than scientific fact. Speaking to some of the UK's most senior and experienced aromatherapists certainly does not give any conclusive verdict. The entire subject is a maze of claim and counter-claim, none of which is help-ful to anyone, except perhaps the lawyers.

Most women during pregnancy run scared of any contact with essential oils, which is a shame when they can be so beneficial at this special time. As a researcher (and mother of four) the best that I can do is to present the evidence as we know it and leave it to the ind-ividual to make her own decisions based on the current knowledge available. As research in this area is ongoing, I recommend looking at some of the excellent websites for further specialist reading. I have listed details for some of the best I have found in the Useful Resources section on p.207. I will also be including information on my own website in the future, as this is an area that has long been of special interest.

The commonly perceived view is that many, if not most, essential oils should be avoided during all stages of pregnancy. For example, the renowned aromatherapist Julia Lawless takes the traditional view repeated in most consumer guides. Writing in her excellent *Illustrated Encyclopaedia of Essential Oils*, she states:

> During pregnancy, use essential oils in half the usual stated amount, because of the sensitivity of the growing child. Oils which are potentially toxic or have emmenagogue properties (i.e. stimulate the uterine muscles) are contra-indicated. These include ajowan, angelica, anise star, aniseed, basil, bay laurel, calamintha, cedarwood (all types), celery seed, cinnamon leaf, citronella, clary sage, clove, cumin, fennel (sweet), hyssop, juniper, labdanum, lovage, marjoram, myrrh, nutmeg, parsley, snakeroot, Spanish sage, tarragon and thyme (white).

She further advises that peppermint, rose and rosemary are best avoided during the first four months of pregnancy. In addition to these, I have also come across researchers who caution against the use of rosemary and all spice oils such as ginger and coriander. Personally, I have yet to discover any clinical evidence that confirms the danger of using any of these oils during pregnancy in a normal aromatherapy context. Indeed, quantities of peppermint oil will be consumed daily by anyone, pregnant or otherwise, who cleans their teeth twice a day with toothpaste – not to mention any pregnant woman with a requirement for minty indigestion remedies or a passion for Polo mints. Several common pharmaceuticals, that have undergone stringent safety testing to obtain a medicinal product licence use very high levels of essential oils and are not contra-indicated for use during pregnancy. For example, Olbas inhaler stick is a pure plant remedy based on inhaling high levels of essential oil vapour directly into the system, including 20 per cent cajuput, 20 per cent eucalyptus and 20 per cent peppermint essential oils. Likewise, the best-selling Vicks VapoRub contains camphor, eucalyp-tus, turpentine, nutmeg, cedarwood and thymol, yet need not be avoided during pregnancy and is even recommended for the skin of babies over six months of age. Similarly, many of these supposedly 'dangerous' oils are eaten with everyday foods such as basil, cinna-mon, clove, cumin, fennel, ginger (a renowned natural cure for morning sickness), nutmeg, rosemary …

Continuing the argument against the scare-mongering approach taken by many aromatherapists is the medical herbalist and leading essential oils researcher, Martin Watt. He categorically states, 'Almost all of the claims made in aromatherapy books about not using certain oils during pregnancy are unfounded.' This is because the toxic effects of some plants in very high quantities were originally based on soluble herbal extracts taken internally, not essential oils used in massage. The only essential oils Martin Watt suggests restricting during pregnancy are birch and wintergreen, as their main chemical constituent may be absorbed by the skin. Neither essential oil is commonly used in aromatherapy. Clary sage, he says, is perfectly safe in a normal pregnancy, but he advises that it is avoided by anyone with a history of early miscarriages.

Essential oils can indeed be very useful during pregnancy and the safest oils for the expectant mum are generally recognised to be chamomile, geranium, sandalwood and citrus oils. Rose is also recommended by some for use after the first trimester. The danger of using rose before then is not clear – presumably we should also avoid all perfumes containing rose oil and give up eating Turkish delight for the first three months? The respected aromatherapist Patricia Davis says she uses lavender in her massage blends from about the sixth month and suggests geranium to help relieve puffy ankles or lemon in a 2 per cent dilution to help venous and circulatory problems. Anyone who has the slightest concern about using essential oils during pregnancy should talk to their G.P. or an aromatherapist who is well-researched on the subject. If you are pregnant, or suspect you might be pregnant, it is also worth telling your aromatherapist before beginning any treatment. Don't forget that aromatic baths are one of an expectant mother's simplest home-spa luxuries and so shouldn't be forgone. Simply choose an essential oil with gentle, skin-caring properties and ensure that the bath water is not too hot. Essential oils are safe to use in skin care blends from reputable companies but, again, remember that even common ingredients can sometimes cause allergic reactions. This is especially true during pregnancy when hormonal changes can trigger increased skin sensitivity. So, my advice is to find a few essential oils that give you real pleasure, run a warm bath, lie back and enjoy them!

fats and oils:
the inside story

Here's a look at how fats and oils break down into their various elements.

Fats, Oils and other Greasy Things
↓
Fatty Acids (87%) + Glycerine (13%)
↓
Saturates + Monounsaturates + Polyunsaturates
↓
Omega-3 + omega-6

All edible oils and fats come under the biological description of 'lipids' and are largely composed of fatty acids with small amounts of glycerin. They are all 100 per cent fat and have around 160 calories per tablespoonful. While they all look much the same, however, there is one small chemical characteristic that makes a vast difference to our health. The fatty acids themselves are large molecules made up of long chains of carbon atoms. Fatty acids vary in structure and may be saturated or unsaturated. In chemical terms, the carbon chains that contain their maximum number of hydrogen atoms are said to be saturated, while those that have less than the maximum number of hydrogen atoms are said to be unsaturated.

There now follows a brief chemistry lesson: all fatty acids have a hydrocarbon 'backbone' made up from carbon atoms strung together like beads. The length of the chain varies from 4 to 26, though the common fatty acids have 12–18 carbon atoms in the chain.

○ Short-chain fatty acids have less than 12 carbon atoms in their backbone
○ Medium-chain fatty acids have 12–18 carbon atoms in their backbone
○ Long-chain fatty acids have over 20 carbon atoms in their backbone

In addition, each mid-chain carbon atom can have up to two hydrogen atoms attached to it. If a hydrogen atom is missing, a double bond is created in its place. These double bonds give the fatty acids their different benefits.

○ 'Saturated' fatty acids have no double bonds (they are fully saturated with carbon atoms)
○ 'Monounsaturated' fatty acids have one double bond
○ 'Polyunsaturated' fatty acids have more than one double bond

The chart opposite shows the pathways of the long-chain (polyunsaturated) essential fatty acids. Figures such as 18:3 beneath each arrow show the number of carbon atoms (18) with their number of double bonds (3). Although both families are similar, they have important differences. However, both groups of fats need the same set of enzymes to work properly, so it is the *balance* of the ω-3 and ω-6 fats that is often so important, not just the quantity.

THE METABOLIC PATHWAY

omega-3 fats

↓

Alpha-linolenic acid (ALA)
Found in flax, walnut,
rapeseed and soya beans
18:3, ω-3 (ALA)

↓

Eicosapentaenoic acid (EPA)
Found in oily fish, cod liver
oil, and small amounts
in chicken and eggs
20:5 ω-3 (EPA)

↓

Docosahexaenoic acid (DHA)
Found in fish oils, marine algae,
and small amounts in organ
meats such as brain,
kidney and liver
20:5, ω-3 (EPA)

omega-6 fats

↓

Linoleic acid (LA)
Found in sunflower, sesame
and safflower oils
18:2, ω-6 (LA)

↓

Gamma linolenic acid (GLA)
Found in evening primrose,
borage (starflower) and
blackcurrant seed oils
18:3 ω-6 (GLA)

↓

Arachidonic acid (AA)
Small amounts are available in
the diet from eggs and meats
20:4, ω-6 (AA)

technical information

OMEGA-6 (ω-6) OIL CONTENT AND STABILITY

Plant oil	Average iodine value	Average ω-3 content	Average GLA content
Coconut (*Cocos nucifer*)	9		
Babassu (*Orbignya oleifera*)	16		
Cocoa butter (*Theobroma cacao*)	37		
Palm (*Elaeis guineenis*)	52		
Macademia (*M. ternifolia*)	78		
Olive (*Olea europae*)	84	1%	
Castor bean (*Ricinus communis*)	86		
Avocado (*Persea gratissima*)	87	1%	
Rapeseed (*Brassica napus*)	92	6%	
Hazelnut (*Corylus avellana*)	94	1%	
Peanut (*Arachis hypogaea*)	94		
Meadowfoam (*Limmanthese alba*)	96		
Argan (*Arganisa spinosa*)	98		
Almond (*Prunus dulcis*)	101	1%	
Apricot kernel (*Prunus armeniaca*)	105		
Pistachio (*Pistacia vera*)	105	2%	
Peach kernel (*Prunus persica*)	106	1%	
Cottonseed (*Gossypium barbadense*)	107		

Corn (*Zea mays*)	115	1%	
Pumpkin (*Cucurbita pepo*)	120	2%	
Wheatgerm (*Triticum vulgare*)	127	6%	
Soyabean (*Glycine max*)	130	7%	
Sunflower (*Helianthus annuus*)	131		
Grapeseed (*Vitis vinifera*)	135	1%	
Poppyseed (*Papaver spp.*)	136	3%	
Passionflower (*Passiflora incarnata*)	138	1%	
Safflower (*Carthamus tinctorius*)	142		
Blackcurrant (*Ribes nigrum*)	143	12%	16%
Borage (*Borago officinalis*)	147	21%	
Walnut (*Juglans regia*)	150	8%	
Evening Primrose (*Oenothera biennis*)	155	9%	
Gold of Pleasure (*Camelina sativa*)	155	35%	
Hemp (*Cannabis sativa*)	166	19%	2%
Rosehip (*Rosa spp.*)	173	39%	
Flax (*Linum usitissimum*)	180	63%	
Echium (*E. plantigeneum*)	190	30%	10%

OMEGA 3 (ω-3) CONTENT IN FISH

Fish rich in long-chain ω-3 fatty acids
Recommended intake: 2–3 grams per week

Type	average grams per 100g serving
Mackerel (raw)	2.5
Mackerel (canned)	2.0
Salmon (raw)	2.3
Salmon (canned)	1.8
Salmon (smoked)	1.1
Herring (raw)	2.0
Herring (Kipper)	2.2
Herring (pickled)	1.5
Sardine/Pilchard (raw)	2.2

Sardine/Pilchard (canned in tomato sauce)	1.7
Rainbow trout (raw)	1.2
Tuna (raw)	1.6
Tuna (canned in water)	0.3
Crab (raw)	0.8
Lobster (raw)	0.5
Cod (raw)	0.3
Coley (raw)	0.2
Haddock (raw)	0.2
Plaice (raw)	0.1

By comparison:

Butter	0.1
Grilled chicken	0.06
Roast beef	0.04

Fish contains more EFAs when eaten raw, hence the healthy Japanese passion for eating sushi. Cold-water fish contain higher levels of protective oils, for example, salmon, trout, mackerel and tuna.

Sources: McCance & Widdowson; US Dept. Agriculture; The Food Commission; *The Good Fish Guide* (2002, Marine Conservation Society)

VITAMIN E IN VITAL OILS

Source (unrefined	*Level mg/100g (average)*
Wheatgerm oil	119
Argan oil	62
Sunflower oil	49
Olive oil	32
Safflower oil	40
Corn oil	21
Peanut (groundnut) oil	19
Rapeseed (Canola) oil	17
Soya bean oil	15
Palm oil	9

weights & measures

g	grams
mg	milligrams (one thousandth of a gram)
ug	micrograms (one millionth of a gram)
ng	nanograms (one thousand millionth of a gram)
ppm	parts per million
ppb	parts per billion
ml	mililitres (one thousandth of a litre)
<	Less than
>	Greater than

glossary

Absolute The aromatic essence extracted from a plant using solvent extraction.

Alpha-linolenic acid An essential fatty acid from which the remainder of the omega-3 (ω-3) family of fatty acids are made.

Arachidonic acid One of the omega-6 (ω-6) family of long-chain polyunsaturated fatty acids. Can be obtained from the diet or created in the body from linoleic acid

Chemotype Varieties of a plant that appear to be identical but which produce different essential oils with differing properties, for example thyme and cedarwood.

Docosahexaenoic acid (DHA) One of the omega-3 (ω-3) family of very long-chain polyunsaturated fatty acids. DHA can be obtained from fish oils in the diet or it may be created in the body from alpha-linolenic acid.

Eicosapentaenoic acid (EPA) One of the omega-3 (ω-3) family of long-chain polyunsaturated fatty acids. EPA can be obtained from fish oils in the diet or it may be created in the body from alpha-linolenic acid.

Eicosanoid Biologically active substance created from fatty acids such as EPA , DHA and arachodonic acid which are produced by cells in tiny quantities. Ecosanoids control many processes within the body, especially those regulating inflammation and the immune system.

Epidermis The outer layer of skin, also known as the stratum corneum, which consists of dead skin cells. Beneath this lies the dermis.

Essential fatty acid (EFA) A fatty acid that cannot be made within the body and so must be obtained from foods in the diet.

Linoleic acid An essential omega-6 (ω-6) fatty acid. The family of ω-6 fatty acids are all derived from linoleic acid.

Lipid Another word for fat.

Lipidic barrier An oily, slightly acidic protective layer that lies on the surface of the skin.

Monounsaturated fatty acid A fatty acid with a hydrocarbon 'tail' that contains only one (hence 'mono') link between carbon atoms in its structure.

Percutaneous By diffusion through the skin, as opposed to subcutaneous which means by injection through the skin.

Peroxides Toxic particles that form as a result of oxidation (for example, after deep-fat frying). High levels indicate that the fat or oil is unstable and more likely to become rancid.

Polyunsaturated fatty acid (PUFA) A fatty acid with a hydrocarbon 'backbone' that contains more than one link between carbon atoms in its structure. PUFAs are described as being 'unsaturated' as they contain less than their full amount of hydrogen atoms.

Precursor A 'parent' substance from which other substances can then be made.

Psoralen Also known as furanocoumarin, commonly found in cold-pressed (expressed) citrus oils and associated with increased photosensitivity with exposure to UV light. Most citrus essential oils are steam-distilled, so are furanocoumarin-free.

Retinol The technical name for vitamin A – a fat-soluble vitamin that occurs in foods of animal origin, notably milk products, egg yolk and liver.

Saturated fatty acid A fatty acid that has its full amount of hydrogen atoms.

Sebum An oily substance secreted by the sebaceous gland that reaches the skin's surface through small ducts leading into the hair follicles. Sebum provides a naturally oily film over the skin's surface that slows down the evaporation of water.

Stroke A common cause of death or disability that occurs when a blood clot or broken blood vessel causes a sudden loss of brain function. Most strokes are caused by a blood clot or extreme narrowing of a blood vessel (artery) leading to the brain.

Trans fats Food processing creates artificial *trans*-fatty acids. These differ from the healthier, natural *cis*-fatty acids and interfere with the way in which the essential fatty acids work within the body. The double bonds in the molecule of an unsaturated fatty acid can be in two forms, either *cis* or *trans*. The *cis* bonds create a 'kink' in the backbone, unlike the *trans* bonds, which allow the molecule to lie in a straight line. In order to work properly in the body, a fatty acid must have all its bonds in the *cis* form. If these are heated to high temperatures, they can flip over to form *trans* bonds. In the body *cis* and *trans* are like a right- and left-handed glove: they look similar but only work one way around. The *cis* form are broken down by the body into useful nutrients, whereas the *trans* form actively prevents this healthy conversion process from happening. In the long term, this means that eating too many *trans* fats can lead to a lack of important essential fatty acids.

Triglyceride The main way in which fat is stored in the body. A triclyceride consists of three fatty acids linked to glycerol.

useful resources

GENERAL CONTACTS

Equazen
Useful essential fatty acid reference website and details of the Equazen range of nutritional supplements, including Eye Q liquid and capsules used in the children's ADHD medical trials. Website includes a quick and easy self-check essential fatty acid deficiency quiz. Highly recommended.

Website: www.equazen.com

The Fish Foundation
For further information on the benefits of fish oils, copies of abstracts and research papers, visit this excellent, regularly updated website.

Website: www.fish-foundation.org.uk

Flora Health
Not the margarine, but the website for the manufacturers of various excellent dietary supplements, including Udo's Choice blended oils.

Website: www.florahealth.com

General Nutrition Centres (GNC)

UK chain of health shops stocking wide range of nutritional supplements and essential oils. Useful website for mail order.

GNC Head office
Nisaba House
Waterfront Business Park
Fleet Road
Fleet
Hampshire GU13 8QT
Tel: +44 (0)870 608 2905
Website: www.gnc.co.uk

Higher Nature

Good mail-order catalogue that includes several useful oil supplements, including Udo's Choice, and CLA shape and weight management supplements.

Tel: +44 (0)1435 882880

International Society for the Study of Fatty Acids and Lipids (ISSFAL)

An excellent membership organisation for doctors, nutritionists and anyone with a specialised interest in this area.

PO Box 24
Tiverton
Devon
EX16 4QQ
Tel: +44 (0)1884 257547
Fax: +44 (0)1884 242757
e-mail: rayrice@issfal.org.uk

Peter Lapinskas

Leading specialist on GLA-containing oils, notably evening primrose and borage oil. Excellent, informative website for anyone who would like to learn more about this area of nutritional science.

Website: www.lapinskas.com

Lipid Library

Run by the Lipid Analysis Unit, grown out of the long history of lipid research at the Scottish Crop Research Institute. The majority of information on this excellent website is on oils and fats analysis. A good free reference and library service for all dietary enthusiasts.

Website: www.lipid.co.uk

Liz Earle Naturally Active Skincare

Botanically-based skincare rich in plant oils, natural-source vitamin E, herbs and essential oils. Renowned for those with sensitive skins. Mail order newsletter and retail stocklist information available from:

Liz Earle By Mail
PO Box 50
Ryde
Isle of Wight PO33 2YD
Tel: + 44 (0)1983 813914
Fax: + 44 (0)1983 813912
Website: www.lizearle.com

The Marine Conservation Society

For details on how to buy fish from sustainable sources contact this environmental lobby group at:

9 Gloucester Road
Ross-on-Wye
Herefordshire HR9 5BU
Tel: + 44 (0)1989 566017
Website: www.mcsuk.org

Marine Stewardship Council

A non-profit organisation that aims to reverse the continued decline in the world's fisheries, by using consumer purchasing power encouraging eco-labelling within the industry.

Unit 4 Bakery Place
119 Altenburg Gardens
London SW11 1JQ
Tel: + 44 (0)20 7350 4000
Fax: + 44 (0)20 7350 1231
Website: www.msc.org

Martins Seafresh

A friendly and reliable family-run Cornish fishmongers with a reliable UK next-day delivery service. Wide range of most fish and shellfish, prepared to order, including traditional and some exotic.

Website: www.martins-seafresh.co.uk

PharmaVita Psoriasis treatment

PS-98 Dermanova Cream

Specific moisturising cream containing fish oils, available from selected health shops or by mail order from PharmaVita.

Tel: + 44 (0)20 8870 5533

Roche Vitamin Information

This helpful source provides specific information on fish oil supplements.

Heanor Gate
Heanor
Derbyshire DE75 7SG
Website: www.vitaminfo.com

MEDICAL SUPPORT ORGANISATIONS

The following organisations can provide further information and support for many of the medical conditions mentioned in this book.

Arthritis Care
18 Stephenson Way
London NW1 2HD
Website: www.arthritiscare.org.uk

Arthritis Research Campaign
Copeman House
St Mary's Court
St Mary's Gate
Chesterfield
Derbyshire S41 7TD
Website: www.arc.org.uk

British Dietetic Association
5th Floor Elizabeth House
22 Suffolk Street
Queensway
Birmingham B1 1LS
Website: www.bda.uk.com

British Heart Foundation
14 Fitzhardinge Street
London W1H 4DH
Website: www.bhf.org.uk

British Nutrition Foundation
High Holborn House
52-54 High Holborn
London WC1V 6RQ
Website: www.nutrition.org.uk

Digestive Disorders Foundation
3 St Andrews Place
London NW1 4LB
Website: www.digestivedisorders.org.uk

Dyslexia Research Trust
Excellent website and support organisation
Website: www.dyslexic.org.uk

Family Heart Association
7 North Road
Maidenhead
Berkshire SL6 1PE
Website: www.familyheart.org

National Childbirth Trust
Alexandra House
Oldham Terrace
London W3 6NH
Website: www.nctpregnancyandbabycare.com

National Eczema Society
Hill House
Highgate Hill
London N19 5NA
Te: +44 (0)20 7281 3553
Fax: +44 (0)20 7281 6395
Website: www.eczema.org

Psoriasis Association
Milton House
7 Milton Street
Northampton NN2 7JG
Tel: +44 (0)1604 711129
Fax: +44 (0)1604 792894

AROMATHERAPY AND ESSENTIAL OILS CONTACTS

Aromatherapy Organisations Council

A governing body for the aromatherapy profession in the UK, composed of aromatherapy associations and a School's Forum. Can supply lists of members, including details of the many professional associations, and further information.

The Secretary
PO Box 19824
London SE25 6WF
Tel: +44 (0)20 8251 7912
Website: www.aoc.uk.net

Aromatherapy Trade Council

Initially formed under the Aromatherapy Organisations Council umbrella and now a separate body representing the British aromatherapy essential oil trade. Remains the UK's authoritative body for the essential oil industry both in the UK and other countries.

The Secretary
PO Box 387
Ipswich IP2 9AN
Tel: +44 (0)1473 603630
Website: www.a-t-c.org.uk

Complementary Healthcare Information Service – UK

Useful resource centre for many complementary therapies, including aromatherapy. Detailed descriptions of many holistic techniques, together with directories for practitioners and courses, including guidelines on what to look for.

Website: www.chisuk.org.uk

Convention on International Trade in Endangered Species of Wild Fauna and Flora (CITES)

Find out more about preserving our rarer plant extracts from this excellent website.

Website: www.cites.org

European legislation

The legislation governing the sale of essential oils and all food supplements continually changes and new guidelines will inevitably be implemented during this book's lifetime. The latest up-dates can be found on the main European parliament website. The news section is good to scan regularly if you are in the industry, while the legislation files provide free searches for specific plants and products.

Website: www.Europa.eu.int

International Federation of Aromatherapists

The longest established international aromatherapy organisation and a registered charity.

182 Chiswick High Road

London W4 1PP

Tel: +44 (0)20 8742 2005/6

Website: www.int-fed-aromatherapy.co.uk

International Fragrance Association (IFA)

Useful collection of research data regarding essential oils and other fragrance materials.

Website: www.ifraorg.org

Martin Watt

A qualified Medical Herbalist and essential oils researcher with an interesting and informative website detailing latest research. Specialises in toxicity studies and dispelling myths within the aromatherapy industry.

Website: www.aromamedical.com

Research institute for Fragrance Materials (RIFM)

Formed in 1966 by the fragrance industry to carry out research on ingredients. A non-profit organisation with useful information on essential oils. Their subsidiary website is the Fragranced Products Information Network.

Website: www.fpinva.org

ESSENTIAL OIL SUPPLIERS

Aqua Oleum

Well-established essential oil mail order supplier run by the aromatherapist Julia Lawless. Stockist of over 100 essential oils, flower
waters and carrier oils.

Unit 3 Lower Wharf
Wallbridge
Stroud
Gloucestershire GL5 3JA
Tel: +44 (0)1453 753555
Fax: +44 (0)1453 752179
Website: www.aqua-oleum.co.uk

Aromatherapy Associates

Well-established aromatherapy treatment centre and own excellent
essential oil product range available by mail order.

68 Maltings Place
Bagleys Lane
London SW6 2BY
Tel: +44 (0)20 7731 8129
Fax: +44 (0)20 7371 9894
Website: www.aromatherapyassociates.com

G Baldwin & Co

Well-established herbal supplier, stocking a complete range of
herbs, tinctures, essential oils and carrier oils. Free catalogue with
more than 3000 different products. Shop open Monday to Saturday
and mail order service. Useful website with option to search by
botanical name.

171-173 Walworth Road
London SE17 1RW
Tel: +44 (0)20 7703 5550
Fax: +44 (0)20 7252 6264
Website: www.baldwins.co.uk

Essentially Oils

Well-established mail order company supplying a very wide range of essential oils (including organically-grown), unusual carrier oils, floral waters, containers and accessories. Useful monthly newsletter sent free of charge.

8–10 Mount Farm
Junction Road
Churchill
Chipping Norton
Oxfordshire OX10 6NP
Tel: +44 (0)1608 659544
Website: www.essentiallyoils.com

Fragrant Earth

Principally suppliers to aromatherapists. Good selection of high-quality essential oils (including organically grown) and ancillary items including floral waters, books, charts, bottles, jars and a good range of essential oil diffusers. Useful regular newsletter sent free of charge with details of regular training courses and seminars, including specialised aromatherapy massage and essential oil chemistry.

The Fragrant Earth Company Limited
Orchard Court
Magdalene Street
Glastonbury
Somerset BA6 9EW
Tel: +44 (0)1458 831216
Fax: +44 (0)1458 831361
Website: www.fragrant-earth.com

Neal's Yard

Reliable retail range of essential oils and some carrier oils. UK shops and mail order service available.

Neal's Yard Remedies
15 Neal's Yard
Covent Garden
London WC2H 9DP
Tel: +44 (0)20 7627 1949
Website: www.nealsyardremedies.com

NHR Organic Oils

Mail order service for high quality certified organic and wild grown essential oils and ancillary items (including handmade aromatherapy chocolates). This company donates 10 per cent of its taxable profits to Action Aid and Friends of the Earth charities.

10 Bamborough Gardens
London W12 8QN
Tel: +44 (0)20 8746 0890
Website: www.nrh.kz

further reading

HEALTH

Fats that Heal, Fats that Kill – the complete guide to fats, oils, cholesterol and human health (1996, Alive Books, Canada) by Dr Udo Erasmus

Smart Fats (1997, North Atlantic Books, California) by Michael Schmidt

Know Your Fats: the complete nutritional primer for understanding the nutrition of fats, oils and cholesterol (2000, Bethesda Press) by Dr Mary G Enig

The LCP Solution – the remarkable nutritional treatment for ADHD, Dyslexia and Dyspraxia (2000, Ballantyne Books, New York) by Jacqueline Stordy and Malcolm J Nicholl. Also available from the Dyslexia Research Trust website at www.dyslexic.org.uk

Phospholipid Spectrum Disorder in Psychiatry (1999, Marius Press) Edited by Profs. Malcolm Peet, Iain Glen and David F Horrobin

The Madness of Adam and Eve (2001, Bantam Press) by Professor David Horrobin. The neuroscientist's view on essential fatty acids and their link evolution and the rise in depression and schizophrenia.

The Good Fish Guide (2002, Marine Conservation Society) by Bernadette Clark. The ultimate consumer guide to eating 'eco-friendly' fish. Highly recommended for every household.

BEAUTY

Perfume and Flavour Materials of Natural Origin (1982, Steffen Arctander's Publications) by Steffen Arctander.

The Illustrated Encyclopedia of Essential Oils (1995, Element) by Julia Lawless.

Advanced Aromatherapy (1998, Healing Arts Press) by Kurt Schnaubelt, PhD.

The Antimicrobial Properties of Essential oils (2000, Winter Press) by Dr Pauline Hili

375 Essential Oils and Hydrosols (1999, Frog Ltd) by Jeanne Rose

Essential Oil Safety (1995, Churchill Livingstone) by Robert Tisserand and Tony Balacs

index